Helping the Stork

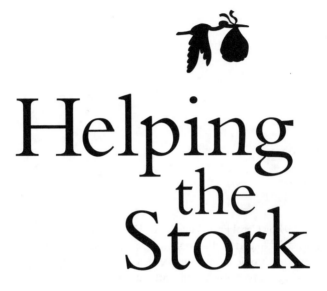

Helping the Stork

The Choices and Challenges of Donor Insemination

Carol Frost Vercollone, MSW,

Heidi Moss, MSW,

Robert Moss, Ph.D.

Hungry Minds, Inc.

Hungry Minds
909 Third Avenue
New York, NY 10022

Library of Congress Cataloging-in-Publication Data
Moss, Heidi.
   Helping the stork : the choices and challenges of donor insemination / Heidi Moss,
Robert Moss, and Carol Frost Vercollone.
       p.   cm.
   Includes bibliographical references and index.
ISBN 0-02-861917-X
   1. Artificial insemination, Human—Popular works.   I. Moss, Robert.
II. Vercollone, Carol Frost.   III. Title.
RG134.M67   1997   97-20535
618.1'78—dc21   CIP
Printed in the United States of America
10 9 8 7 6 5 4 3

Book design by Rachael McBrearty—Madhouse Productions

Contents

Support for donor conception is invaluable, as grateful readers of Helping the Stork's first edition let us know. Now we are grateful to our editor at IDG Books, Stacy Collins, as well as to our editor on the first edition, Betsy Thorpe, who was with Macmillian when publication moved ahead too suddenly to add our sincere thanks! We also appreciate the persistence of our agents Shelley Roth and Ellen Denison who believed *HTS* could be a classic though not a blockbuster bestseller!

One trend since *HTS* first was published is increasing online resources, which we've tapped to keep readers updated. Our web site offers updated links for organizations and news of interest to DI families, at: http://members.home.net/mossre/stork.htm. You can email us at cfverc@world.std.com, mossha@juno.com, or mossre@home.com, or write to Carol at 29Cedar Ave., Stoneham, MA 02180.

Bod and Heidi keep a low profile locally, respecting their children's privacy. They prepared *HTS*'s first edition by writing a story for their son and daughter about DI. Soon afterward, her daughter said thoughtfully to Heidi, "So, Daddy has asthma and I don't. That's because I don't have his DNA, right?" She was only six — but she'd grown up with Bob preparing biology lectures! Every few months, she makes a comment like "the donor guy must have had freckles." Their son never raises the topic, reflecting that each child — and parent — reacts differently to donor conception.

We're glad *HTS* can offer many more families, as well as their loved ones and medical teams, well-deserved support.

—*Carol, Bob, & Heidi, June 2000*

A Note on Terminology

L anguage has its limitations. We fall into shorthand terms, like "DI family," rather than longer, more accurate phrases, such as "a family whose child was conceived with the help of donor insemination." We've also created some new terms, such as "wide-open parents." No family fits any simplistic label. We hope our language won't distract you from the support and guidance we've intended.

For our contributors, we will be using first names only, unless someone is professionally or publicly involved in DI and wishes to use his full name. Contributors may or may not have chosen to use their actual first name. We're deeply grateful to the dozens of people who wrote of their experiences, and to the hundreds who taught us over the years what DI is all about.

We've tried not to censor people's quotes, even when their terminology or views would be upsetting to some readers. People's raw feelings are important to express, especially given how voiceless those involved with DI have been.

To avoid saying "his/her" every time we want to refer to a child, we'll refer randomly, we hope equally, to each sex.

When we refer to whether a child is or isn't biologically, genetically related to her parent, we will often refer to a biological or nonbiological child. We don't wish to denigrate the status of the child's origin. All children, no matter who is parenting them, have the same origin, a biologically normal one of an egg and a sperm forming an embryo.

The majority of people considering DI are married couples with no sperm or impaired sperm. This is the group with which the authors have the most experience. We hope single women can overlook our use of "couples" when the information applies just as much to unpartnered women. We hope lesbian couples can translate information for dads-to-be when it is as true for the nonbiologic mom.

We frequently use tentative words, *might, somewhat*, and *maybe*. We've done this deliberately, to acknowledge that all situations and people are not the same. We believe that what we are saying applies in most cases, but want to be respectful of those whose ideas and experiences differ.

We welcome your comments. And please let us know if your feedback, experiences, and suggestions can be used for future articles or revisions to this book.

Introduction

The longing for a child can be one of the most powerful in life. Anything that threatens to leave that dream unfulfilled can be devastating. When you must consider family-building alternatives, the choices can seem overwhelming.

Donor insemination (DI) is one alternative that is widely considered. It offers the chance for medical treatment that can be relatively low-tech, with little delay and much less expense than either adoption or high-tech medical alternatives such as in vitro fertilization (IVF). DI is very often successful, offering the chance to experience pregnancy and parenting a healthy newborn.

DI has been practiced in the United States for over a century, widely since the 1950s. This was tied to increased legal protection of all parties involved: the doctor who located a fertile man willing to provide his sperm, the "donor" who was paid a nominal fee to emphasize that he retained no parental rights, and the married couple who chose to use sperm from a donor.

By the 1980s, many more men were learning that their hopes of fatherhood would require either DI or adoption, and adoption had become much more difficult and costly. Also at this time, unmarried women without children, whether single, divorced, or in lesbian relationships, began to seek out doctors willing to help them to become mothers via DI. The awareness of the danger of sexually transmitted infection increased the use of sperm banks, where sperm was frozen and quarantined until the donor could be repeatedly tested.

The actual medical procedures involved in DI can be simple. Parents-to-be usually work with a gynecologist who specializes in fertility treatment to pick a donor, to pinpoint ovulation, and to decide what techniques of insemination offer the greatest chance of achieving a pregnancy. Some ask a friend or relative to donate sperm, to become a "known donor." Some women prefer to use donor insemination without the assistance of a doctor, in the privacy of their own home, using simple home insemination techniques.

But many women must seek out an infertility specialist. Their gynecological problems require that donor sperm be linked with some of the more high-tech, costly medical procedures of reproductive endocrinology. And DI doesn't work for everyone, a sad ending after months of alternating hope and frustration.

The secrecy that surrounded donor insemination in its early decades lingers today and creates added barriers for those searching out resources and support. Nevertheless, help is available as a couple considers DI, picks a medical team, selects a donor, makes medical decisions during the treatment, and as they parent. This book is the first to pull together the input of consumers, as well as professionals from medical and counseling backgrounds, to offer objective guidance through each stage of the DI experience. Many readers may need to pore over every page before they can even consider DI as a pathway to parenthood. Some may decide to head back to other alternatives, including further medical approaches, adoption, or living without children. But we hope this book can provide reassurance that there are many ways to successfully build a family with DI.

If you are considering using donor insemination, it may be comforting just to learn that you're not alone. Thousands consider donor insemination each year, often unsure where to turn for information and support. *Helping the Stork* can help you break through that isolation. Throughout the book, you'll hear from many others who have gone down these paths, whose experience can help you envision how your family will meet DI's challenges. We'll start with our experiences.

BOB'S STORY

I was working at the part-time job I had taken as a computer consultant at a New York financial firm to supplement my teaching salary, saving for the baby we expected to be expecting. The owner's secretary looked concerned. "Your wife called. She wants to meet you outside the building. Is everything OK? She sounded hysterical."

What could I say? I certainly didn't want my client worrying about my personal life. How about "We've been trying to get pregnant and my wife is getting some test results today and we're probably not able to have children"? No, that wouldn't do. "Everything's fine. My wife's just a bit emotional." That sounded better. I headed for the sidewalk.

Despite New York's impersonal reputation, I noticed people stopping and turning to watch as a woman ran hysterically down the street, crying out loud. I grabbed the crying woman as she ran toward me and put my arm around her, thinking I had to be strong. "It's OK, it's OK. Calm down. Shhh. I can't understand you."

Sounds like a novel? Unfortunately, it was painfully real. If you've had to deal with male infertility, you've almost certainly experienced similar pain. From the day of the diagnosis of my infertility, I decided my job was to be strong and not to think about the implications of what we were doing. I pushed on, never looking back—from finding out on that terrible day in 1988 that I had nearly no sperm, through the decision to do DI, through the roller-coaster ride ending in failure each month, and through testicular cancer in the middle of it all.

While some agonize over the DI decision for months, I approached the problem quite logically and unemotionally (at the time).

> My count was too low for in vitro fertilization with 1988 technology.

Heidi wanted the experience of pregnancy.

We would know one biological parent, who would contribute half of our child's genes.

We would control our baby's prenatal care.

We could parent a newborn, not always possible with adoption.

For us, everything came down on the side of DI.

We were so anxious for a baby, we couldn't wait until we knew what we were doing before we jumped in. We began inseminations, and only after we'd begun did I realize that I hadn't addressed my emotional concerns, and perhaps the toughest was grieving the loss of my biological "dream child." My two really positive traits that I clearly imagined sharing with my child were my intelligence and my thick, curly hair. While they are quite different sorts of traits, these are the two I had hoped to pass on! It may sound superficial to those who haven't gone through this mourning, but remember, most of us have held these images for decades. Having a child who might have little in common with my mental picture was a difficult prospect for me to face.

The other major emotional issue for me was the inequality between my wife's contribution to our babies and my own. Would our kids naturally have a stronger bond and relationship with her? Would the kids reject me once they knew I wasn't their biological father? This remained a major source of insecurity for years. It has largely gone away now that I see how much I love my kids and they love me, but it does linger as a fear of future possibilities.

Five months into trying, these concerns began to look larger than life, and I became discouraged because we weren't pregnant. I was fed up and wanted a child. NOW.

As a backup plan to our efforts with insemination, we began investigating adoption while also urging our physician to step up the medical efforts. But in our seventh cycle, we finally tried IUI (insemination directly into the uterus), and that month we finally became pregnant! All of our friends, not knowing about our use of DI, said, "See, you weren't infertile, you just had to relax." We nodded in agreement and smiled, as our doctors had suggested.

Once we were pregnant, we figured that all of the DI issues would disappear. But they didn't. We talked and worried more about these issues during our pregnancy than while we were doing DI. Not until our perfect little son was born did infertility stop being the major focus of our lives.

HEIDI'S SEARCH FOR SUPPORT

Twelve months into trying to get pregnant the old-fashioned way, I found myself walking into a doctor's consulting room to learn the results of a postcoital exam. I had set up the initial tests with an infertility specialist, carefully choosing a woman, whom I thought would be less intimidating than most male doctors and more understanding.

But even before I could sit down, the doctor coldly delivered the news—my husband didn't have enough sperm to get me pregnant. Bob could try seeing a urologist, but it probably wouldn't help. The doctor advised adoption or "adopting a sperm" if we wanted children and showed none of the compassion I had been looking for as she cavalierly demolished my dream of our perfect biological child. In tears, I ran out of the room—and never went back.

When I sobbed out the news to Bob on that Manhattan sidewalk, he seemed to take it stoically and went back to work. I was surprised and didn't know how he could work if he was experiencing nearly as much pain as I was. I needed to talk with someone, to share my pain. As soon as I got home, I called a therapist I'd just begun seeing due to our difficulties starting a family. She said not to worry, at least there was no problem with me! I still have no clue why she thought that was a comforting thing to say. It seemed like I'd always have to be alone with this pain.

But to my surprise, Bob came home an hour later. I thought he could push it all aside, but I was wrong. Although he did manage to hold it all in for a while, a few days later Bob's tears were flowing with mine. Our infertility bond began and made our next year bearable.

We did decide to have Bob see a urologist, and even before the doctor began his workup, he told us to keep any results a secret and to "untell" whatever we had already said to family and friends. He warned us that if we decided to use a donor, we wouldn't want anyone to know. It made sense at the time, so we told everyone who knew of our problem that Bob would be OK with some treatment and we would probably be able to have children.

I am not the type who can handle problems without the support of family and friends. Bob was very understanding of my needs, and together we decided that it would be OK to tell my best friend the truth, so I wouldn't feel like I was lying to her on a daily basis. At that time, as far as Bob was concerned, she would probably be the only relative or friend ever to know. I was also beginning the search for others who had been through DI, sure that this would help us cope and relieve our feelings of total isolation.

The doctor we saw next had a counselor in the office to meet with couples beginning DI. She helped us understand some of the basic medical issues, but offered no other support—except to advise secrecy. She then chose our donor, trying to match Bob's appearance from the small selection of donors at that practice's own bank. We seemed ready to get started because we didn't know any other options existed to be explored. If we had done DI any differently, we would not have our uniquely wonderful son and daughter, an unthinkable possibility.

Our family is now complete, but our understanding of DI continues to deepen. I have wanted to help couples with DI ever since finding out for myself how little support and information are available. During our own experience we had felt like pioneers, breaking new ground. Of course, we weren't, with an estimated 30,000 babies born via DI each year. But with secrecy so complete, we seemed to be totally alone, even in a city where there must have been thousands of others going through the same pain. I started the DI hotline for the RESOLVE of New York City (a local chapter of the national infertility organization providing support, education, and advocacy). I decided to get a master's degree in social work while caring for our first baby, so I could begin a career in infertility counseling.

We decided to write this book to help other families cope with the ups and downs of the DI process. The openness of this action has certainly crystallized our decision about when to tell our children about DI and about being "wide open" with the truth behind our children's conception. We long ago told our families about our use of DI and have been laying the groundwork for helping our son and daughter meet their own challenges, though it may be years before they fully understand DI's meaning in their lives.

CAROL'S PERSPECTIVE

In my years as an infertility counselor, I've heard many powerful stories of families responding to DI's challenges. In 1979, when I began to set up services for infertile couples through RESOLVE's national office, I was beginning my own saga with female infertility and felt empathy with the loneliness of male infertility. I wanted to help couples turning to donor insemination find support, but most couples weren't ready to "come out of the closet." So my first group for couples considering DI met in 1982 on a first-name basis, an option that still helps many attend even today. A wonderful couple who were trying for their third child volunteered to come and speak, and the pictures of their adorable daughters brought tears and reassurance to the group.

I continued my commitment to DI families into my years of private practice and in my volunteer work with RESOLVE. Offering workshops taught me how reassuring it is for newcomers to learn from others, and how much parents can gain from sharing their wisdom. It has been wonderful to see people find a safe, accepting place to celebrate their successes and share their inside humor, as well as voice their concerns. I'll always remember Janet, who had kept DI so private, attending an especially large "Trying Times" meeting and saying in amazement, "This feels like a party!" The message that DI can be a joyous way to parent seemed to be lost in books and articles that tried so sincerely to raise possible problems for parents-to-be to consider. I wanted to pull together possible solutions as well. Any wisdom I've been able to pass on in this book comes from years of listening to the experiences of the many families who've shared their joy as well as their pain.

If you've been all alone with your experiences with DI, we hope this book will encourage you to reach out to others and to find at least a small inner circle of confidants who can come to understand its challenges in your life. Don't go it alone!

Chapter One

Family Building:
DI as an Option

In my sixth grade autograph book, where it says "What I want to be when I grow up," I listed "Scientist." I was intrigued by the mysteries of life, how a single cell, the fertilized egg, becomes such a complex creature, a you or a me.

My parents bought me a small microscope. I loved to look through it at all sorts of things. When I went through puberty at the ripe old age of fourteen, of course I wanted to see sperm. And I did. Just once. It was neat, seeing these little things swimming around, carrying my genetic information.

A few years later I tried again. I prepared a slide, placed it on the microscope, and focused—nothing, almost no sperm. I didn't know what to make of it. Perhaps I'd done something wrong. I just passed it off, put it aside.

I always wanted to have children, and I was even more impatient to have them than Heidi was. Years later it was Heidi's gynecologist who confirmed what I think I'd known deep down, since my second slide. I was going to need quite a bit of help in realizing my dream of fatherhood, and I'd have to adjust that dream—just slightly. I would have all those great parenting experiences . . . except experiencing the genetic connection, which is a bit of an irony, given my career as a biologist.

—Bob

"Be fruitful and multiply" is a powerful phrase, both a commandment and a promise from God. It's seen as the purpose of life for men and women, central to marriage vows, to perpetuate the species while creating a visible symbol of their love for each other. Society celebrates the joys of pregnancy and the rewards of parenting.

People who want to become parents make assumptions about what it will take to get there. Many expect difficulty in finding a life partner with whom they'll happily parent. Many worry about how they'll afford children or how good they'll be at parenting. But few expect that just getting a baby conceived will become their major problem.

When the longing for children is threatened, it's *not* a minor issue. Even those who have been ambivalent about parenting don't want their choice taken away. Having your own baby seems so easy for the fertile world, something taken for granted. Those who can't fulfill that goal often feel defective, inadequate, or guilty at letting down their partner and their families. Many feel angry, wondering "Why me?" Many fall into depression, finding that their sense of purpose in life has become unclear.

For the families who contributed to this book, babies didn't arrive easily. Some of them had lots of warning—they were cancer survivors or men with vasectomies not easily reversed. For others, however, the inability to easily have kids came as the biggest surprise of their lives.

Although this book focuses on donor insemination, we aren't pushing DI as an easy solution. Rather, we want to give donor insemination the in-depth, objective, and respectful attention it deserves. When we first put out word that we were writing this book and asked for contributions, people wrote from around the country. Many of them stated that the difficulties of DI were well worth facing because DI brought a uniquely precious child into their lives; they couldn't imagine loving any child more.

We also want to give voice to those for whom DI didn't work. Some who considered DI decided instead to adopt or persisted in trying for a genetically shared pregnancy. Some moved on without adding a child to their family of two. Our focus is on finding a resolution that works for you. *Resolution*, the term from which RESOLVE draws its name, evokes the often slow, painful process of resolving the emotional crisis of childlessness while finding the resolve to make choices about your remaining options.

AN INTRODUCTION TO DONOR INSEMINATION

Controversy still surrounds donor insemination as well as other forms of "third-party reproduction" or "collaborative reproduction," such as surrogacy and egg donation. DI isn't as socially acceptable as adoption, even though it's almost as common. While people can be insensitive about adoption, few would make remarks as blunt as "That's disgusting" or "I could NEVER do THAT!" Patricia found the lack of encouragement striking.

> I cannot remember anyone saying, "Great, I am so excited by that opportunity for you," as I think they do when told of adoption plans. Unlike adoption, where usually everyone knows someone who has been touched by it, people don't know that they have been touched by DI because no one will admit it.

The newer alternative of egg donation has a more positive reputation, with egg donors viewed as brave, generous young women wanting to help sad, childless couples. When society turns to DI, jokes and smirks break out. Both infertile men and donors are fodder for comedy, as demonstrated in the movie *Made in America*. As one DI mom succinctly put it, "DI involves masturbation and ejaculation. If there were a sad, painful way to get the sperm, it might be more acceptable." The lack of social acceptability greatly reduces people's confidence in telling others and makes parents want to protect their child from possible ridicule.

Throughout *Helping the Stork*, we'll look at why DI has been such a well-kept secret. This is confusing for anyone beginning to learn about

DI. There must be something terribly wrong if it's so little discussed, right? Involving the help of a third person to provide sperm is seen by some as going too far to have babies. Many DI parents, donors, and even medical practitioners would rather avoid subjecting themselves to negative judgments, and parents are certainly protective of children. So you probably don't realize that donor insemination is very common or that you may already know a family who turned to DI, but if they knew you would respect their choice, they'd probably share their experience. Our commitment to confidentiality for the contributors in this book has given dozens of families a chance to offer their words of wisdom.

DI parents are often amazed that anyone expects them to be as open about their child's conception as adoptive parents are urged to be about their child's arrival. They feel adoptive parents are open because they must be—a baby suddenly arrives without a pregnancy. Heidi was stunned that everyone who'd known of Bob's problem assumed without question that some miracle of modern medicine had "cured" him—or that she had finally relaxed enough to get pregnant. When DI parents do try to tell loved ones of DI's role in their pregnancy's beginnings, they're often told, "Oh, you don't need to be so open!" For DI, unlike adoption, couples need to make deliberate decisions about disclosure.

The relative ease of keeping DI private has also kept families isolated. Those considering DI or getting started with it have had difficulty finding answers to their questions or providing information for their family and friends, the inner circle we focus on in our next chapter. This is starting to change as there is greater openness.

Not everyone considering DI views it through the lens of male infertility. Men who have survived cancer, spinal cord injury, or chronic illness may be thankful to even be able to consider parenting. If they've survived a traumatic or life-threatening situation and been able to move on to the planning to have a child, DI may seem to offer more opportunity than loss. Men who want to spare their children a genetically transmittable illness can be glad DI exists. Couples with vasectomies may find stepfamily concerns more difficult than the complexities of DI itself. Unmarried women and lesbian couples may be delighted to have an option allowing them to plan thoughtfully for a pregnancy. The experiences that bring you to DI will affect your choices and challenges.

MALE INFERTILITY: NEWS YOU NEVER EXPECTED

A diagnosis of male infertility leads couples to medical realities they never imagined facing. Men with absolute infertility often find their hopes ending brutally and quickly; despite advances in reproductive medicine, many men learn that their type of infertility is untreatable, given the medical technology available to them. In contrast, men with impaired fertility watch their hopes slowly die over years of advanced treatment with low odds and high costs.

A semen analysis often brings the news. This test can be humiliating, enraging, heartbreaking, and only ruefully funny in hindsight when talking to others who know what it feels like not to do well on one of the most important exams of your life. As one man joked, "I didn't study and scored a big zero." Because gynecologists focus on women, they tend to overlook male infertility, medically and emotionally. Diana remembers her gynecologist's mistake when reporting Jeff's first semen analysis.

> The doctor read his results to me over the phone; they were normal. We kept trying. Several more months passed and I decided to switch doctors. I went to pick up my records. I perused them as I walked down the medical building hallway. I came across the sperm test results. The number of sperm detected was 0; motility, 0. There were no sperm detected. I don't remember the details of how or where I told Jeff. I specifically recall the two of us sitting on the bathroom floor, a towel over both our heads, hugging and sobbing. Later I got a letter of apology from my gynecologist.

Sometimes there's a forewarning—for example, if an earlier post-coital test found no sperm or if some past event led a man to suspect infertility. Sal echoes the thoughts of many men in saying he wondered why there had never been a surprise pregnancy in all his single years of imperfect contraception. George remembers being ill with the mumps during puberty.

> I had mumps when I was at camp, and my brother wrote a long letter to my mom with a short note at the end about my mumps. It was the family joke for years; here I was suffering with a huge swelling in my testicles and it was just an afterthought for my brother. When I found out about my infertility and traced it back to the mumps, the story of my brother's letter home was never mentioned again. A family joke had turned into a forbidden subject.

Some men know their medical history is no joke. They were aware of their infertility before marrying but perhaps harbored hope that there would be treatment available in time. Single men who know they're infertile wonder when to raise this topic in a new love relationship. Liza remembers:

> Tom told me that he was sterile the first night we slept together (in response to the usual question about using birth control). By this time I was too emotionally committed to him to back out and thought that I would be able to deal with the consequences down the road. Obviously I didn't have much hope of processing this piece of information on the spot!

Some men blurt out the news too early, before the relationship can withstand the impact. A man may long for reassurance that this woman will stick by him, that childlessness will be fine. A woman may need the reassurance that there's some way they can become parents if they marry. Two upset people may end a relationship in distress at this disclosure stage. If a man withholds the information for too long, in denial, too ashamed, or too defensive, she may feel betrayed and misled.

For most couples there's no warning, and the news is a brutal shock for both. As one man wrote, "Without any sensitivity, this doctor destroyed all my hopes and dreams."[1] One woman went in to see her gynecologist alone, thinking they'd go over her early test results; when the doctor asked if she was sure her husband had ejaculated, she knew they were in trouble. It's normal to assume there must be a lab error, as few people are aware how common male infertility is. Protective denial comes in to cushion, or at least delay, the blow. However, confirming the semen analysis may be more suspenseful. Marie and Ed got a letter after the first analysis saying Ed's sperm count was "extremely low," but they assumed the repeat test would be fine. With the second letter they learned he "had absolutely no sperm. Not one. The cause unknown."

Men with such drastic news often undergo more tests. Hormone levels can indicate whether testicular tissue that's supposed to produce sperm cells has shut down. Blood cells can be karyotyped to see if a chromosomal problem, such as Klinefelter's syndrome, has caused infertility. Physical examination of the testicles can give clues to the cause and extent of the damage. A biopsy of the testicles can show if sperm cells stopped maturing or if there's an operable blockage. Sperm, if present, can be surgically extracted for in vitro fertilization (IVF) with a micromanipulation technique such as intracytoplasmic sperm injection (ICSI). Even though high-tech intervention is available, it requires women to go through an extensive medical process to produce and then retrieve multiple eggs to maximize the chances of these laboratory procedures' succeeding. A husband often feels guilty when his wife goes through so much because of *his* medical problem. A wife may feel angry, especially if her effort is minimized by a husband who is defensive. She may also feel guilty if she's reluctant to go through IVF or discouraged about the chances for success.

For men with better semen analyses, whose fertility seems to be only impaired rather than destroyed, the same alphabet soup of options may apply. The results of multiple semen analyses can vary widely, so the prognosis may look good one time and bad the next. Even when a man has seen an andrologist (a urologist specializing in male infertility and reproductive endocrinology), he might not have definitive answers to his questions. Male infertility research lags far behind female, and controversies abound. Roger's sperm morphology appeared to be OK according to the older method of analyzing sperm shape, but when fertilization failed during an IVF cycle in the early 1990s, a new method was used, the Kruger or strict morphology analysis. Roger remembers, "I went from being OK to being sterile, overnight!" Some specialists say only an IVF cycle can test whether the sperm can fertilize eggs.

Many men get results that at first they don't understand to be bad news. After all, societal wisdom says, "It only takes one sperm"—if only that were true! It may take months for some medical professional to explain that the results really aren't so great. A shared pregnancy might be possible only with an incredible expenditure of time, money, and effort, and there are no guarantees. Emily and Patrick dealt with this scenario.

> "It only takes one sperm," my doctor reassured me every time I went for another intrauterine insemination, until my last visit, when she suggested I move on to IVF. It had been over two years and we were realizing that our dream of having children was becoming just that, a dream.
>
> It was then that my husband went for varicocele surgery [to treat a varicose vein in the groin, often associated with male infertility for reasons that are not well understood]. We patiently waited six months to see if the surgery had made a difference. There was a slight improvement, but not enough to achieve any fertilization on our second IVF attempt.

Some men terrify their wives because they react *too* well to their diagnosis. "These things happen, and if I can't have a child of my own, we'll figure out what else we can do" might just be denial, a temporary pushing away of anguish. But for some men this reaction reflects a long-standing attitude toward life. They choose not to ask, "Why me?" or "What could have caused this?"—questions that can torture others. Instead, they accept the loss and shift to practical solutions and other ways to get kids. These men should be gently encouraged to express their loss but shouldn't be told their approach is wrong.

Some men know they aren't OK. Interviewed in *In Pursuit of Pregnancy*, Eric touches on common themes.

> It's not that Lisa wasn't involved or supportive, but I couldn't really explain to her what my male feelings were. I never thought I'd be macho about it, but I really was. I always assumed that it would not be a problem with me if I had a fertility problem, that I would want to do the most plausible thing—adopt. I hadn't even considered the possibility of AID [the old term, artificial insemination donor]. Thank God I had my shrink! My lifelong dream—to have a family—was so important to me for as long as I remember, and now it seemed an impossibility.[2]

Some feel their masculinity is threatened, even though they may wonder why they feel that. Some feel terrified that friends or relatives will find out and ridicule them—which happens more to infertile men than women. Some men are flooded with a sense of inadequacy, wondering why their wife would stay with them. Some shift from insecurity and shame to defensive anger, rejecting all offers of medical intervention or emotional support.

Men may find it difficult to mourn their biological child. Even those who have carried a clear mental picture of that child may not easily express their loss. They may feel bad acknowledging they've longed for a child who would share their interests, talents, and abilities. Of course, a biological child can be quite different from the one a would-be father has pictured, but infertility forces a man to completely abandon that picture, cold turkey, with a tough withdrawal period.

Men don't have to mourn alone, but they may find it so stressful to see their wife's reaction that they wish they could. For many men a wife's feelings about infertility cause more pain than their own. If the wife is more driven toward parenthood, it can be terrifying for a man to realize that his medical news deprives her of her dream, creating a baby together. His guilt at putting her through this experience isn't rational, since male infertility is rarely caused by something he did or didn't do. Yet that makes the emotion no less powerful. Stephen asked Connie, "If you'd known this about me before we were married, would you have married me?" Her answer, while jarring, was honest, "If I'd found out while we were just dating, I would have stopped dating you. I would never put myself into this situation on purpose." Connie explains:

> I was on the verge of a breakdown, or so I thought. It seemed like I had gotten married and now I was digging my grave. There was nothing more to live for. All my dreams were shattered, and there was no way to get them back. This was happening in the spring and summer, and I don't remember ever seeing any sun. At that time it didn't matter that he was a loving person and would be a loving father, because he could never be the father of my children anyway. Fortunately, we stayed married, because I do have a loving husband who was able to see light when all I saw was darkness.

A wife also faces the reality that her dream child will never exist. She married her husband assuming his best qualities would someday be reflected in their children. Heidi and Bob joke that she married him for his beautiful hair and his ability to make great chocolate chip cookies and that he can pass on at least one of his best features! But it took a long time and a lot of communicating to get to this point of joking. For some couples there's so much overwhelming loss and despair that the difference between healthy grieving and depression becomes unclear. Women often want to put pain into words, an approach many men are less comfortable with.[3] Both can feel very alone with their grief. Leigh remembers: "We found out after a year of no birth control. We really were devastated. Having been together for about eight years at that point, I felt that we were so close to each other, yet at that moment so far away too."

Often the pain and the decisions are too overwhelming to face with only each other for support and guidance. A couple's usual mechanisms for connection, from sharing news of their day to making love, can be overshadowed by the intensity of this crisis. Sherry writes, "The impact of my husband's infertility on our sex life was immediate and devastating. Overnight, sex became a futile exercise that served only to remind us of what we could not achieve."[4] Many infertile couples seek out counseling for the first time in their lives.[5] An objective person can help bridge differences in perspective, helping a couple feel connected and committed to getting through this challenge together.

INFERTILITY AS A SIDE EFFECT: MORE THAN AN INCONVENIENCE

For many men the inability to have a biological child is actually secondary to another health problem that is often far more threatening than the resulting infertility. A list of illnesses affecting reproduction would be extensive, but three are so common—cancer, genetic disorders, and spinal cord injuries—that they are discussed separately below. The losses resulting from any serious or chronic illness present ongoing emotional issues. To add infertility to these can deepen or reactivate a crisis.

Sometimes the damage to fertility occurred so early in a man's life that only a pediatrician or parent might have realized it. The doctor may have minimized or avoided the topic of future infertility, viewing the parents as already distraught over their child's illness or treatment. The illness's connection to infertility may not have been understood at the time. If the man's parents were informed but withheld the information from their son, he and his wife might understandably be furious when they finally learn that infertility could have been predicted.

No matter how a couple learns of an illness's impact on the husband's fertility, short-term counseling can help. She is now suffering the impact of his illness too. For both of them, his infertility and their option of DI is a huge readjustment of their dreams for pregnancy and parenting.

Cancer's Effects: Glad to Be Alive, But . . .

The most frequent illness that leads its survivors to DI is cancer. As cancer survival rates rise, so do the numbers of men getting to the stage of marrying and wanting children. Chemotherapy devastates sperm production, as does radiation in the area of the testicles. Some surgeries, especially for testicular and prostate cancers, can impair the nerves causing erection or ejaculation.

Even if a patient is told of fertility effects, it's not unusual for him to block out or minimize the news. A man may be too preoccupied with fighting his disease to let the concept of infertility sink in. "It will never happen to me" is a common form of protective denial. "I'll never want kids anyway" is another version for young men who years later realize the emotional impact. Many physicians don't deal with the "side effect" of infertility, feeling they have already overwhelmed their patient with bad news. Some oncologists believe the patient must focus on cancer survival, on accepting treatment regimes. But talking about family building can be an affirmation that there will *be* a future, important for loved ones too. Adolescent or adult cancer patients should be urged to self-bank sperm before treatment, one of the first purposes of sperm banks. In one Massachusetts court case, *Harkness vs. Children's Hospital*, the patient won a malpractice suit because his oncologist didn't advise him to bank his sperm before cancer treatment.

Some men learn of their infertility during their diagnosis or treatment for cancer. Dan and Lisa got doubly shocking news soon after their honeymoon.

> In May of 1986, Dan was diagnosed with testicular cancer. We'd only been married about four months, so we hadn't even seriously discussed having children. The doctor told him then that he might want to bank some sperm, but the bank found a zero count. I was really naive, having just turned twenty-one. I told them I'd have Dan come back to give more. "That won't be necessary, your husband is sterile." The longer I look back on that phone call, the more angry I get with the way they broke the news to us.

Many men never bank their sperm. Often they are so frightened and overwhelmed by the cancer that they can't handle arranging for banking. For younger men, freezing sperm can seem too weird or unimportant. A teenager might not even be comfortable discussing masturbation, let alone sperm banks. Many of these men or their wives are later tortured by regrets, wondering if their samples would have been excellent, if pregnancy might have been possible. It can be very hard to let go of regrets.

Some men who do self-bank later find it to have been a futile effort. Well, not exactly—many say the hope alone was invaluable, especially if they were already in love and planning to parent. Hope may have fueled them through months of cancer treatment and, later, inseminations with their frozen sperm samples, which in turn may have prepared them for inseminations with donor sperm. Bob Levin writes about adopting, but his words ring true for donor insemination as well.

> I don't remember if he actually used the word sterility. He probably did, doctors always preferring the formal term, hiding behind it. . . . And leaving the stunned patient to do the plain speaking: You mean I won't be able to have kids? EVER? What I do remember is how upset I was, and how surprised at being upset. I had cancer, after all; I could hardly complain if the drugs that were supposed to save my life also had some unfortunate side effects. And besides, I'd never thought much about having kids. I was 19. . . . There was a visit to a sperm bank, a hedge against a future time when some baby-making imperative might suddenly seize me. . . . Some 15 years later . . . my wife and I sent for those frozen specimens . . . a bad omen that, as they came out of the deep freeze, a few of the specimens self-destructed—their container exploded, is what I was told . . . black humor.[6]

Some couples feel they can't cope with parenthood during their years of greatest anxiety about recurrence of the cancer. Others want to get pregnant quickly, as an affirmation that he'll survive or to give her a child to love and care for if he doesn't. The biological deadline for a wife's fertility may mean that pregnancy is now or never. Bob and Heidi decided not to wait because his testicular cancer was diagnosed when they were already six cycles into DI. As Bob recalls:

> After my initial surgery, our therapist suggested we put off trying to get pregnant. For most people that would have been sound advice. Obviously there were a lot of emotional adjustments to the cancer diagnosis. But once I learned my cancer wasn't likely to be fatal, the diagnosis only made me more determined to have children as soon as possible. I wasn't going to let the cancer keep me from my goal of having a family. We continued with DI and were pregnant a month after my surgery. Only one astute biologist friend counted back from the due date and inquired how Heidi could possibly have gotten pregnant merely one month after the removal of my cancerous testicle. My reply? "It just goes to show . . . it only takes ONE!"

Genetic Disorders: A Fresh Start through DI

For men with genetic disorders, trying for a pregnancy may not carry the joy it might have otherwise. Whether to risk passing on their genes is a difficult and personal choice. While the decision is easier with diseases as terrible as Tay-Sachs, what does a couple do if the disorder is less devastating? What if the genetic risks are unclear or the disease might soon become treatable? A genetic counselor can help sort this out, but ultimately this tough decision will be the couple's.

Some men carry genes for genetic disorders for which prenatal tests are available, such as sickle cell anemia (a blood disorder), cystic fibrosis (a respiratory and digestive disorder), and fragile X syndrome (a cause of mental retardation). In these cases couples can opt to conceive using their own sperm and egg and turn to prenatal diagnosis to help them avoid genetic transmission. Another option is preimplantation testing, that is, using IVF laboratory testing before implanting only embryos free of the genetic defect. Genetic tests are available only for some disorders, although more are announced every year. Scientists are just beginning to understand the inheritance of most illnesses, including cancers and mental illnesses. The statistical risks of passing on many diseases, such as schizophrenia, are impossible to define because the causes aren't understood. Given these considerations, turning to a donor with a healthy genetic background may be a better option.

Some men may not be aware of the risks of passing on their condition. Physicians sometimes minimize or avoid discussing the risks of genetic transmission. No doctor wants to make a patient feel more "defective" or limited by emphasizing the effects his disease could have on his children. The patient, his family, and his medical team may feel that advice not to reproduce robs him of his own sense of self-worth. It's hard to look objectively at what to do for the next generation, especially if a man is still making sense of the impact on himself.

A special concern for couples with genetic illness is the genetic history of their chosen donor. It's hard to trust that a donor knows his genetic history thoroughly. Couples can share their concerns with sperm bank staff, who can spend extra time going over a potential donor's medical history. Those who turn to DI because both partners are carriers of a recessive genetic disorder, such as Tay-Sachs or cystic fibrosis, will of course want to know their donor has been tested.

Spinal Cord Injury: Disabled but Able to Be a Dad

Another group of men now living on to become dads are those whose ability to father a child is impaired by spinal cord injury (SCI). Many more people today remain healthy because of increased understanding of the preventive-care needs of paraplegics and quadriplegics. Increasingly, men with SCI have the confidence to marry and plan to have a family.[7] A National Spinal Cord Injury Association fact sheet states the case well.

> One common misconception following a spinal cord injury is that a single man or woman will never find a life partner, or that an existing partner will leave a relationship due to the complications of an injury. This is not

the case. The divorce rate following spinal cord injury is only slightly higher than in other populations, and thousands of people have been married and begun families after a spinal cord injury.[8]

Men with spinal cord injury may try for a pregnancy using low-key vibratory techniques or high-tech IVF approaches. Some couples head straight to donor insemination. No matter what, family and friends may be surprised to learn of their family-building attempts. If they haven't yet adjusted to the man's disability, they may not view him as ready to become a parent. This assumption alone may be so infuriating that he doesn't even attempt to explain DI. It can be tremendously helpful to talk to other dads dealing with similar physical limitations, as well as with other DI dads.

Vasectomy Effects: Starting over Again

For couples facing the effects of vasectomy, it can be frightening to approach donor insemination from such differing perspectives. The husband is trying to begin a new family, which may be stressful if the previous family experience was an unhappy one. The wife, most often childless, longs to have her husband's baby. Without successful reversal, the dream of creating a "mutual child" is dashed.[9] Clyde writes:

> I felt a pregnancy in my second marriage would be a mere formality of reversing my vasectomy, resting a few weeks, and getting "back in the saddle," so to speak. I was rudely awakened . . . after finding I was "spermless" as the very procedure [IUI] was about to occur. I was shattered! Not only did I feel inadequate, but I had failed at the very moment, the only medically required moment, when I HAD to do my part.

Some vasectomy reversals do work, and men who are considering this option should consult skilled specialists, although paying out-of-pocket for reversals or IVF with surgically retrieved sperm may not be feasible. Yet many find it hard to let go of their only hope, however slim, for a genetically shared pregnancy and view DI as a last resort. For others

DI is an easy choice, so much so that reversal surgery doesn't seem worth high costs or low odds.

No matter what leads them to DI, men often blame themselves for making the vasectomy decision or for having blind faith in reversals. They may feel guilty that their choice in the past is so deeply affecting their new wife now.

A wife may blame herself—for marrying someone who'd had a vasectomy, for being the motivating force behind the failed reversal, or for wanting a baby so badly. Anger is inevitable, and a common target is the first wife, who got to have his children, usually still has custody, and may have pushed for the vasectomy as the "fairer" contraception choice. Elizabeth writes:

> I felt angry and jealous that my husband's ex-wife was able to have his biological children and I never would. I felt she was lucky to have his children, didn't take care of them, and left her marriage. I could never have anything she had, including my husband's desire to have a family.

Grief can be very deep for women who fear they'll always be stepmoms but never moms, especially if stepparenting has been difficult. Her family and friends may blame him for taking away her chance to be a mother.

These couples knew from the beginning of their relationship that they'd have added challenges. Both partners need to stay in touch with their belief that their marriage can withstand all the stepfamily stresses. They deserve to know that they aren't alone in taking this leap of faith in a future family.

Single Women: Last Call for Pregnancy

When a woman isn't in a committed relationship but longs to be a mom, turning to DI is often the most difficult option. It's controversial enough to consider motherhood without a husband, but to do so via a sperm bank or with a friend's gift of his sperm may seem just too unconventional. It's wise to set aside final consideration of any options until she has fully grieved the loss of most women's first choice, the often lifelong dream of sharing a pregnancy with someone she loves. As one woman writes:

> Sadness arises from a feeling that I am giving up on doing this in the traditional way. Envy of others who have it all. Unbearable sorrow that there is no intimate love relationship in my present. I have a need to fully accept this so that I can let go of it and make way for the joy that can follow.[10]

For many heterosexual women, the dream of "Mr. Right" includes love, marriage, and the baby carriage, in that order. Many women work toward that goal, but it doesn't arrive before they find that time is getting tight. Peggy writes:

> I think that for most people DI is a second choice. I know it was for me. My first choice would have been to marry and to have my husband provide the sperm to enlarge our family to include a child. I never married but I believed that my biological clock was winding down and I wanted to become a mother before it was too late. I wanted to have my own biological child.

Choosing single motherhood has become an option as more women have achieved financial independence and as lifelong marriage has become a much less easily achieved goal. Yet to go ahead into the most permanent job of her life without a partner can be terrifying. That so many women are considering it is testimony to the powerful rewards of motherhood. If the baby carriage does come first, this doesn't at all rule out love or marriage in a woman's future. But it certainly changes her immediate future.

In addition to DI, some women consider other options, such as asking a friend or former lover to help with conception "the old-fashioned way," conceiving with his not-fully-aware help, adopting, or becoming involved with nieces and nephews. Some of these options may seem easier than DI, but each has potential disadvantages too.

Women becoming moms on their own can draw on the wisdom of Single Mothers by Choice. This organization went nationwide in the 1980s as the media spread word of meetings in New York begun by Jane Mattes, a psychotherapist and single mother. Her 1994 book, *Single Mothers by Choice*, draws on all she has learned from listening to hundreds of single women considering motherhood, trying to become pregnant, and parenting alone. Single women turning to DI will find guidance in Mattes's book, and attending SMC chapter meetings can be invaluable.

Much of our language focuses on couples, but each chapter offers much for SMCs as well. Women may well feel relieved not to have to hammer out every DI decision with someone else.

LESBIAN COUPLES: TWO MOMS AND MORE CONTROVERSY

Lesbian moms are not new, but the numbers of women choosing to bring children into their relationship represents a growing trend. As lesbian couples have found greater acceptance in society or have created supportive communities, the public act of sharing a pregnancy together has become a viable option.

As with any couple facing a lifelong choice, one member may be more ready and enthusiastic than the other. It's easy to take sides, one arguing for DI, overstating the positives, while the other focuses on the problems. It's important to reach a solid decision, particularly because the co-parenting relationship of two moms may not be as legally protected as that of heterosexual parents. Many lawyers advise drawing up an agreement of intention to co-parent in which parenting plans are clearly defined, to serve as a road map should the future include times when a couple has lost their way.

DI is only one family-building option to consider, and it may not be the easiest to reach agreement on. Although adoption hasn't been easy for lesbian couples, thoroughly exploring adoption options may be a better choice. Some women are stopped cold at the thought of judgmental doctors or intrusive tests. But within the choice of DI, many options exist, and finding an acceptable pathway may be possible. Perhaps only home insemination with the help of a known donor is acceptable. Maybe an alternative insemination program for lesbian couples or the help of a caring medical team is worth traveling some distance for.

When discussing family-building options with family and friends, lesbian couples have to face their reactions. Obviously, if DI is leading a woman to come out to a friend or family member, there might be some added factors in their responses. For family and friends who have long accepted the couple relationship, there may be a new stage of working through the image of a family with two moms. For protective loved ones, there may be fear of society's crazier homophobes. They may need to hear how lesbian moms create boundaries and an inner circle of support. Some family and friends may accept the sexual preference of two adults but believe that it's wrong to subject a child to homophobia or that a child shouldn't be brought into a lesbian relationship. Here, the studies of successful lesbian moms may help reassure them that children can blossom with two moms too. This book and others for lesbian moms may be able to help loved ones understand how DI can be a workable, wonderful choice.

The next chapters will provide information helpful in DI choices, but most of the examples will focus more on married couples, with husbands as the nonbiological parent. So much of the DI "system" developed in the face of the stigma surrounding male infertility. It may not be ideal if a chapter seems overly oriented toward heterosexual couples, but lesbian couples may find it interesting to compare and contrast the issues they're dealing with as they move along this pathway to parenthood.

•

We hope that reading about the many perspectives of those arriving at donor insemination will offer new insights, intellectually and emotionally, no matter what has raised DI as a concern in your life. Finding a way to fulfill your longing for children may seem impossibly difficult at times, but we hope we can offer you support and guidance along your pathway to resolution and, we hope, to great joy in parenthood.

Chapter Two

Facing Tough Choices

The ambivalent couples have such a tough time. They often ask if families I know are happy with DI—"almost always" is true for those who sought help deciding. The more determined, "pro DI" person needs to hear a spouse's pain, and look at the other alternatives. I share what I've learned from wonderful folks who have made their peace and moved on, with and without ever sharing a pregnancy, with and without children.

All human beings like quick fixes, but couples must make DI choices to last beyond their lifetime.

—Carol

Donor insemination can be a wonderful way to bring a child into your family, but before you get to that stage, you must face some tough choices. DI is a highly charged subject, and you'll need to understand the conflicts and controversies that have become a part of it. Unfortunately, the secrecy that has so long surrounded DI makes it difficult even to find the information you need and safe places to discuss how it applies to you. You need an "inner circle" of confidants as you start to learn about DI and later as you live out those choices. Many couples aren't very open as they consider DI; the topic is too painful, and many aren't sure how private they will want to keep their choice of DI if they decide to proceed. You can always be more open later, but for now you must find decision-making support.

SETTING UP YOUR DECISION-MAKING TEAM

If you choose to try for a DI pregnancy, you will eventually have a whole team helping you achieve your goal. Your team will include the staff of the infertility specialist(s) you consult, sperm bank professionals or your known donor, and confidants who offer you emotional support. Your team may also include one or more professionals trained in counseling, who focus in on DI or help you manage other personal or marital issues that might otherwise become overwhelming when the pressures of DI are added in. You may need an advocate if you find you aren't skilled at asking for what you need, especially from medical professionals. Your team may also include contacts from support organizations or peer support groups who can offer the wisdom of first-hand experience and understanding.

Your team will need to remember that you and your partner's needs are the focus of this project and you hold the ultimate vote on if and how to proceed. You should feel free to pick whatever role or position within the team that feels right for you at any given stage. At times you may function as the coach; at other times you may feel more like a rookie in need of lots of guidance. At certain points you'll want to be able to defer to someone else's judgment, to rely on his or her greater skill or experience to guide you through the next step. This team will be most successful if you know how to set your boundaries, asking for help when you need it or indicating that you don't need the help being offered. As you get to know the strengths and limitations of your team members, you will know whom to rely on at each stage.

BECOMING INFORMED ABOUT DI'S DIFFERENCES

DI is not a new family-building alternative, but it has a long tradition of "Don't ask, don't tell." DI involves differences, and differences scare and confuse most people. Few DI parents feel sure that their way of having a family will be widely accepted. As one mom with a toddler puts it, "I just don't want to subject myself to people's ignorance." She joins the many thousands who feel at least a bit guilty for not speaking up in favor of DI, knowing that it can be a very good way to build a family—just different. Most decide it's easier to keep DI relatively private.

You will need to find some way to cope with attitudes about DI. The topic brings up some very strong feelings, even when based on very little knowledge. One man expressed his opinion via the Internet:

> To me artificial insemination is almost like your wife having an affair and getting caught. That may sound sort of crude and demeaning but I consider myself a traditionalist. And using another man's sperm is just like having an affair with him—to me.

Bob has heard similar knee-jerk reactions from students in his biology courses, which each semester cover reproductive technologies. One student writes:

> Our class represents a large variety of cultures, opinions and backgrounds and because no one favors artificial insemination, it draws me to the conclusion that the only people who would use it are those females who wish to be single parents, and female homosexuals. No couples would use the sperm donor method; it seems a crude and unintelligent choice.

DI is caught in a vicious cycle—almost no one doing DI wants to subject themselves to public opinion, so the public keeps drawing its own negative conclusions, lessening parents' interest in speaking up on DI's behalf.

DI is different because it is viewed negatively by a number of organized religions. The most vocal has been the Catholic Church, which has a long-standing doctrine that rejects reproductive technologies of any type. Many Catholics, conservative Protestants, and Orthodox Jews hear from clergy that DI is adulterous because a third party is involved, violating the union between spouses. Another concern is the possibility that two young adults unknowingly conceived with the same donor might marry. DI can cause a crisis of faith among those who ask how the natural, loving, and powerful longing to bear children could be viewed so judgmentally by their religion. Many learn for the first time to turn inward, to examine their own conscience, to formulate their own ethical views.

DI has its own vocabulary of terms that are definitely different, and for some couples this seems to add to the sense that DI is a bizarre way to begin a family. As you read about DI, you'll see the older term "AID" (artificial insemination by donor), which was abandoned when it became confused with AIDS, and "TDI," which adds "therapeutic" to the name. (One mom jokingly wondered if that was intended as a contrast to home insemination, which must be recreational!) "Cryobanks" have "catalogs" of donors, and their "donor managers" help you narrow the list of "profiles" you'd like to read. You can ask a friend or brother to be a "known donor" or a "directed donor." Your medical team can do "ICI" (intracervical insemination) or "IUI" (intrauterine insemination) or move to an "ART" (assisted reproductive technology) cycle. References to family members as "donor offspring" or "social dads" can be especially distressing.

The media highlight DI's differences; talk shows and magazines thrive on controversy. Heidi was told by a TV producer that she and Bob were too happy—no one would be interested in their story. Reporters can do better in portraying DI than the talk shows because they can use pseudonyms, and families are glad to help if they aren't subjecting their family to a total loss of privacy. But genuinely positive pieces of any depth are few and far between, and therefore precious to parents, who save articles carefully for years.

DI affects the people who encounter it differently over time. Many of the issues you face as you consider DI, and many of the stresses you go through in trying for a DI pregnancy, fade with time once you've completed your family. When you first realize that DI may be an option you should consider, you think about it all the time—or expend a great deal of energy avoiding thinking about it. Once you're a parent, DI absorbs very little of your time. Yes, there are peak times, even crisis times, when DI is an issue. But your child is your child, and your daily routine has little to do with who is genetically related to whom. As Marty puts it, "DI might have been difficult if my son wasn't one of the world's ten best kids."

UNDERSTANDING DI'S TRADITION OF SECRECY

Many of your choices about donor insemination will be affected by the secrecy that has so long surrounded it. You may decide that DI isn't the right option for you because its controversies make either openness *or* secrecy look too burdensome. If you do want to proceed with DI, many of the decisions ahead, such as selecting a donor, will flow from your initial thoughts about whether or not you will someday tell your child about it. Couples who struggle with this decision now can hope to feel more at peace as they live out their choices as parents.

DI's first recorded use in the United States is an almost unbelievable story of doctors' taking secrecy for granted. In 1884 an older Quaker merchant and his young wife came to the Jefferson Medical College in Philadelphia because they were unable to conceive. The group of doctors discussing the merchant's sterility decided to help. They voted on the best-looking donor, and without sharing their plan with either the husband or the wife, used this donor's sperm to perform an intrauterine insemination while she was under anesthesia. She became pregnant, and after the birth the physicians confided in the husband—but at his request, never in the wife.[1]

For much of this century, physicians continued to keep DI out of the public eye. The practice of secrecy became institutionalized, accepted as a necessary or desirable part of donor insemination, as the next chapter also details. The traditional approach was to provide very little information about the donor and to suggest that couples tell no one of their experience with DI. As one doctor wrote:

> A state of consciousness has to be achieved in which the donor, from the psychologic point of view, does not exist. Donor semen should be then

regarded as "material" from an anonymous testis, the donor being actually a "nonperson." For this purpose we restrict information given about the donor to an absolute minimum.[2]

DI recipients were almost always couples dealing with absolute male infertility. It was assumed men couldn't face society's attitudes or think about DI's emotional issues. Many obstetricians and gynecologists accepted as a given that any pregnancy was better than adoption or childlessness. It was common to use more than one donor per cycle so that no one could guess the genetic parent. Physicians would carefully destroy records of which couple had been matched with which donor. When June got pregnant in 1960, her doctor made her promise not to tell anyone.

> He said it was breaking the law, it was committing adultery. I said OK, I won't tell and for almost 25 years, other than my husband and my mother, I never told a soul. . . . I am a very honest person. . . . So as the years went by, this became a heavy burden for me. I knew my daughter had a right to know.[3]

This policy of anonymity was a product of the times; there was neither societal acceptance nor legal protection for DI.[4] Physicians feared they'd be sued or shunned in their community and religious groups. They felt that the donors, often their students or junior colleagues, needed protection from the threat of future legal claims and from societal condemnation.[5] Advances like bone marrow transplants didn't even exist; there may have seemed to be little medical need to preserve data on who was biologically related to whom.

But when something *must* be kept a secret, particularly in the opinion of an authority figure like a physician, it's usually assumed that something is "wrong." Donors could not be openly proud of their contribution to creating longed-for families. Dads felt unable to fully proclaim their joy in having a child with whom they shared so many bonds, though not their genes. Mothers felt prohibited from sharing the full story of what they went through to have their precious but sometimes bittersweet experience of pregnancy. Without any way to validate, compare, or reassure themselves, parents could wall off their feelings, often even from each other, and do as they'd been told. Or they could violate the wishes of the physician who had enabled them to become parents, and tell others, knowing there would be painful reactions from many. Whatever choice they made, they went unsupported.

By the late 1970s these beliefs and pressures had begun to shift. In 1981 RESOLVE's founder, Barbara Eck Menning, wrote an article for an ob/gyn journal urging physicians to see the choices about DI as belonging to the patients, not the doctor.

> I think AID [the old acronym, artificial insemination donor] is a piece of information, like adoption, that parents must view as the child's right to know. Considerable risk? To whom? As we develop more professional standards for AID, should we not lessen the obsession for self-protection and increase our concern for the recipient couple and child?[6]

Change was also stimulated by the adoptee rights movement, which challenged any withholding of information as a violation of an individual's rights, as well as the consumer movement in medicine. As sperm banks became more predominant than physician-recruited donors, fears related to protecting a local donor from identification began to fade.[7] "Profiles" began to provide nonidentifying information about donors, giving parents-to-be more information to share with a child.

As we head into DI's second century, much is in a state of confusion. Professionals now differ widely on anonymity for donors and on disclosure to children. The few studies that have been done on this issue show that many families with young children are still keeping DI very confidential, but no studies have tracked families with older children. Physicians voice concerns that the recommendation of greater openness is being made without evidence of children's responses. One family therapist, concerned about secrets, has a different view:

"Physicians profess secrecy to be protected from the complex task of counseling and educating the couple about raising a child with a different genetic parent."[8]

Parents have many differing views on anonymity and openness, but most agree that the decisions about what is best for their families should be theirs to make. The medical community is starting to accept, even expect this, leaving disclosure decisions and donor selection up to the recipients. In the 1980s Karen and Marty were asked by their doctor to get a letter from Carol, their infertility counselor, to attest to their mental health, which was questioned because they had told relatives and planned to tell any child about DI. Now many physicians recommend counseling for couples who find donor selection too distressing or who can't agree on if or when to tell their child. There has been a remarkable change in the practice of DI in a relatively short period of time.

FORMING YOUR EARLY DECISIONS ABOUT OPENNESS

Every DI family faces two major decisions: if or when to tell a child about his or her conception and how private or open to be with anyone else. Of course, these two issues clearly affect each other. It becomes difficult to have shared with a number of loved ones but not with the loved one most affected, your child. So if you are not planning to tell your child, you must keep DI private, with the possible exception of a small inner circle of carefully selected, discreet confidants. If you do tell your child, especially at an early age, then how open you become with others may depend on how open your child is. The decision about privacy may be taken out of your hands when your child tells the story about the nice man with sperm! If your strong preference is to share this only with a small inner circle, then your child's developmental capacity for discretion must guide what and when to disclose. It's always possible to move toward greater or earlier openness than you originally planned. But a decision to be widely open with others or to tell a very young child will commit you to this path.

The term *secrecy,* when used most appropriately, applies to the decision not to tell the person that the information relates to, in this case the child. But the term is often used when referring to maintaining privacy with others.[9] Something secret is thought to be bad, a source of shame; to keep a secret is to be dishonest or to lie. Secrecy in DI is compared to secrecy in adoption, but adoption can only be the worst-kept "secret" around—everyone but the adoptee knows that he or she joined the family in a different way. Many DI parents believe they can and should keep DI private to spare their children pain.

There is no positive term for information kept from a child for protective reasons, with loving motivation. Some professionals, struggling to find a more neutral term than *secrecy,* have tried *nondisclosure.* You need to find the words that express what you believe. But no matter what words you use, sometimes there will be stressful feelings.

Although your disclosure plans may change over time, it can help to picture yourself dealing with children who do or do not know about their conception's special circumstances.[10] Try to imagine not only the stages you think you'll deal with easily but also the toughest tests of your decision. Imagine how you might feel and what you might say when:

> Your child starts asking questions that involve genetics—why he wears glasses or where she got such curly hair.

> Your teenage son's friend is adopted, and your son tells you he's so glad he doesn't have to deal with that.

> Your daughter, a young adult, wants to contact her donor.

These situations may seem frightening now, whether you imagined telling your child or not. They're difficult to focus on if you're still experiencing the unhappiness of childlessness, and you may feel there will be time to fill in the gaps as you go. But coping will be easier if you carefully choose a path and later re-evaluate if it's continuing to meet your family's needs. Images of responding to your child, whether revealing DI or not, will then flow more comfortably. There will be feelings of uncertainty; they just won't be as overwhelming. If you can face these issues, a sense of well-being will be conveyed to your child, even if only in subtle ways.

This comfort with your decision may not come easily. Both discussion and introspection are needed, looking at both the pros and cons. Talking to a counselor or a DI parent can be invaluable but may also force you to hear or read about views you may not want to deal with right then. It's especially tough to be confronted with opinions about the rights of children to know of their DI origins if you can't imagine sitting down for that talk. Hearing from others who are comfortable with their choice can help give you clarity about what's important to you, as well as confidence in your ability to make your own choice.

Any decision must be acceptable to both you and your spouse. Don't just reluctantly acquiesce to your spouse's wishes.[11] At first it may seem impossible, but other couples have worked their way to a shared plan, often with some counseling. If a couple who aren't yet DI parents can't agree on a shared vision of whether or not to disclose DI, then maybe DI isn't for them.

Men often feel that it's easier for the genetically related parent to decide to tell. But women are just as afraid of their child's disapproval and just as protective of their child's vulnerability to society's crueler views of DI. Both men and women fear temporary estrangement from adult children outraged that they weren't told earlier. But women need to understand that men feel afraid of losing their connection with their children permanently. Because moms are still so often the "primary parent," the one a child runs to for comfort, it can be terrifying for a man to risk that his emotional connection is strong enough to reveal that there isn't a genetic connection between him and his child.

Those committed to nondisclosure need to think about any conditions under which they might wish or need to tell. If your child becomes upset by differences in appearance or overhears confusing information about her conception, you might want to explain DI to clear up her concerns. If you can imagine how you'd tell, you may be less afraid of the future possibilities.

Similarly, we'd ask those most committed to disclosure to read about the approaches and attitudes of those not planning to tell. The concepts of reserve, dignity, discretion, and boundaries will hold meaning for any parent who hasn't yet told her child or whose child prefers that the parent not tell others.

PLANNING NOT TO TELL YOUR CHILD

Many people aren't convinced that there are compelling reasons to tell a child about DI or that it's wrong to keep secrets from their child. Almost all couples agree that a poorly kept "secret," one that is known to many others, is unwise. But many parents believe they can keep this secret from their child without damage. In fact, they believe that this is their responsibility, partly because they've heard that this type of information can be so upsetting.

Professionals debate why parents decide not to disclose DI. After questioning a group of parents seen for psychotherapy, Annette Baran and Reuben Pannor, authors of *Lethal Secrets* and advocates for openness in DI as in adoption, concluded that couples are primarily protecting the shameful secret of the husband's infertility.[12] But a study that looked at both men's and women's feelings about donated eggs as well as sperm came to a different conclusion.

> Gender differences exist for disclosure regardless of whether there are eggs or sperm being donated. This challenges the notion that men choose not to disclose only because it may be damaging to their "male ego."[13]

Even if more women than men consider openness, a strong percentage of both moms and dads have no plans to disclose DI to their child.

In our experience talking with couples, protecting the child is usually their primary concern. A parent may be glad to take on public opinion about male infertility or DI, but dread their child being teased on the playground. They don't want to risk that their child will react badly. It's hard to dismiss fears when other bad things (such as cancer, infertility, or spinal cord injury) have already changed your life. Talking with other dads when his son was six, Sean said, "I had a bad enough relationship with my dad, especially as a teenager. I don't want to do anything to jeopardize my chance to have a good relationship with my son." He later decided that their relationship was going so well that he would tell his preteen son, but that was a carefully considered decision.

Parents who choose nondisclosure often see withholding information as sparing their children confusion about their genetic background. Connie and Stephen write:

> We are confident that he will be happy, healthy, and successful in his life. After all, he did come from good genes and has a very loving and nurturing environment. Do we confuse his life with the truth about those genes?

Marie and Ed conceived their twins with the help of his brother, and they don't plan to tell the girls. Their inner circle includes his brother's girlfriend and Marie's closest sister. All feel that very little is being concealed from the twins.

Some couples consider disclosure a form of dumping issues on the child, especially if the child won't be able to get much information about the donor. They fear their child might embark on a futile search or feel obsessed with this difference. Some parents say not telling is putting the painful past behind them. They consider ongoing discussions a self-defeating refusal to get on with life. Even though many parents feel less adamant over time, they then face a new dynamic— they've gone this long without telling and can see no compelling reason to tell now.

If you are deciding to keep DI from your child, you must find ways to deal with any tensions that arise. Keeping information from your child doesn't mean you can just "forget" DI, making it a taboo topic with your spouse. You need to commit to talking to your spouse whenever an issue is on your mind, and listening whenever your spouse needs to talk. If that's difficult for you, a confidential source of outside support can help, someone objective and caring.

No matter how certain you are of the choice not to tell, you will cope best if you can acknowledge that sometimes this decision will have serious disadvantages or challenges. Couples must accept that one of them will be less comfortable than the other. Even the best secret keepers feel bad at times for concealing information or directly misleading a loved one. You need to prepare yourself for the times your child asks you questions you can't answer honestly, questions based on the assumption of shared genes.

There is always the possibility that you'll find nondisclosure can't work for you forever. Larger issues may arise; you may feel ethically bound to tell your child of her origin. One common example is if a dad is diagnosed with a disease that his child might fear inheriting. Knowing there is no genetic connection could save her from anxiety. On a happier note, DI may become so much better understood that you want your child to know that you too chose this alternative and feel it has been a wonderful choice for you.

PLANNING TO TELL YOUR CHILD

The preliminary decision to tell your child someday can be reached for many different reasons and handled in many different ways. Many people are accustomed to openness on other issues, at least with those closest to them. Some people were raised in families with a secret not well handled, an issue they're unwilling to re-enact. Some have read stories about adults who believe that secrecy about their DI origins severely damaged the closeness in their family.[14] In 1992 Bill Cordray was quoted in a *Boston Globe* article that was picked up by other publications nationwide.

"Growing up, I never had any connection with my dad," recalled Cordray. "I had a sense of being psychologically different. . . . And he seemed to be angry all the time. I think now that it was probably anger at having to pretend to be my father." Cordray learned the truth in 1983, a year after his social father died. Despite his sense of distance from the older man, his first reaction was disbelief. "Later, I became resentful," he said. "I believe I could have had a close relationship with my father if it hadn't been for the secret."[15]

Margaret Brown found out at age sixteen after her parents had been divorced nine years and she expressed interest in seeing her estranged father. In college she submitted her opinions for a *Newsweek* column.

To deny someone the knowledge of his or her biological origins is dreadfully wrong. . . . Parents must realize that all the love and attention in the world can't mask that underlying, almost subconscious feeling that something is askew. . . . Future donor-recipient parents must step out of their own shoes and into those of the person they are creating. Parents can choose to raise a child honestly—fully respecting the child's individuality—without the self-imposed pressure to deceive.[16]

Karen and Joseph speak for many in saying, "If we keep DI a secret, it might give our kids the feeling that there is something wrong with what we did, if they ever found out. We can't live a life of lies."

Although many questions about when and how to tell need to be worked out over time, parents like Karen and Joseph plan to eventually share whatever information they have, and expect to support their children in searching out whatever added information they'll need. Of course, "telling" isn't a one-time event. Parents are often unsure how much to tell at any given stage and when they should raise the topic if their child doesn't. But they are committed to learning and tend to take one of three major approaches.

Parents who are *wide-open* are planning to discuss DI from their child's earliest years, gradually adding to their explanations. Some were very comfortable with openness from the time they began considering DI. Tom, who has done media work on DI, writes:

> Neither Joanna nor I wanted to keep secrets during our infertility. It was hard enough as it was. Otherwise, how would we even be able to answer the simple questions from our friends and family: "How are you?" and "What's new?" We didn't want to isolate ourselves; we definitely did want to be comfortable with the topic by the time our baby came. We didn't want to add the burden of our shame to whatever other burden a donor-insemination origin might become to our child.

Some are open because they want to help change the isolation and ignorance surrounding DI. As Tom and Joanna wrote in an article for their RESOLVE chapter newsletter, "Parents help their children most not by hiding, but by standing up to any bias that exists against them and teaching them that bias is the bigot's problem—not theirs." These parents feel that early explanations are best for a child, so that there's a gradual deepening of understanding over time. Erin, trying for a pregnancy, wrote to the *New York Times Magazine* "Letters" (that's open!):

> We are going to be only too happy to have our future child know that its uncle helped us make this "best choice for us." I understand parents wanting to keep potentially destabilizing information from a child. However, there is no stronger bond than the truth.[17]

Once you talk with a five-year-old, you have to be prepared to be wide open. Your child may proudly announce, "My mommy went to a sperm bank!" or "The doctor got a man to help us have my brother." But as Jim puts it, "Dealing with the fall-out from honesty is much easier than keeping track of who knows what."

Parents who plan to keep DI for *loved ones only* are waiting until their child is capable of using discretion in talking about DI. Many parents wait until their child's preteen years, before adolescent conflicts and identity issues but not until she's developed some capacity for understanding DI and for maturely choosing whom she might wish to add to the family's inner circle. These parents have often limited their inner circle, wanting their child to know first. Diana writes, "Our approach at this point is openness with our children and privacy with most others. We tell family members and close friends with whom we feel comfortable." Many children between ages eight and ten, with some guidance and forethought, can join in decisions about sharing this private information. If a child wants to tell someone, he needs to know that it's OK, that he doesn't have to keep a "family secret."[18] Parents will need to explain that DI has been kept private not because it's bad but because it's personal and, among some people, controversial. Many parents have a relative who can't be trusted to be discreet or accepting of DI. Most children will already know what the story is with that relative. *Every Kid's Guide to Overcoming Prejudice and Discrimination* is one good resource, explaining that some people don't form opinions with an open mind, without prejudging.[19] Children also need to know which loved ones have been supportive confidants, which ones know that DI has been a wonderful family-building choice.

Parents who wish to keep DI disclosure *for adults only* plan to tell their child as a young adult because they believe a person has a right to know about his genetic origin but want to be very private when their child is young. Most feel they can better face their child's anger at not being told earlier than deal with the repercussions of earlier disclosure. If a child has to face other difficulties, it may seem to a parent that there's no appropriate time before adulthood, when maturity may bring greater strengths to adjust to this news. Some parents undertake very thorough preparation, such as keeping an ongoing journal about their experiences with DI, to document for their child why their best parental judgment was to wait.

Privacy or Openness with Others

Even if you've disclosed DI to your child, you may face complicated decisions about who else needs to know, now or ever. You need to decide where to draw your boundaries, who will be part of your inner circle, and who has no appropriate place in it. Carole LieberWilkins, who has led groups for parents not biologically related to their children, explains, "You want to be sure you're not assuming you'll keep this private while your wife is telling the delivery room nurse the whole story of your baby's conception!"[20]

Most families who plan to tell their children still have privacy concerns. You don't have to explain how you finally managed to get pregnant or why your child looks more like her mom. You can develop a public "cover story" that reveals only what is appropriate. Couples have pretended that surgeries and in vitro fertilization (IVF) cycles were successful when they never occurred. Many can get away with "You wouldn't believe all the doctors we saw," true with DI as well. Then turn the topic to what you do feel is appropriate to discuss—usually your joy at finally being pregnant or parenting. Andy was often asked, "What finally worked?" and would respond, "Persistence," sidestepping the specifics. David would say, "He's a miracle," the truth after years of trying.

Keeping DI private may cause some feeling of distance between you and your family and friends. Heidi lost a close friendship because she chose to tell very few people of DI until the children were told. Her relationship with her friend went from a comfortable and loving one in which everything was shared to a relationship with limits. This added to the distance created by her friend's lack of understanding and compassion about infertility, and they became just casual friends.

It may be tempting to tell friends even if you don't plan to ever tell your child. Avoid this—it can cause heartache and paranoia over the years.[21] As your child grows older, you may fear he will sense adult tensions about some quickly dropped topic. You may come to avoid certain friends who might "slip" and refer to genetic differences. You may even fear that a former friend could maliciously choose to tell your child about DI or that a judgmental friend could do so "for your child's good." As your child begins to be a participating member of your inner circle of adults, you may feel guilty that she doesn't know about her own background when others do.

WHOM CAN YOU TRUST TO COOPERATE WITH YOUR PLAN?

Most people do indeed confide in at least one trusted friend, relative, or professional. If this person is someone on your medical team or a counselor, confidentiality is routine in their professional lives. If it is a close friend or relative, you need to think about how they in turn will get support in sharing any burden associated with your secret. If you want your sister to support you, she may need permission to tell her best friend, and realistically she must be able to confide in her spouse. You must make realistic assessments before telling anyone and then clear agreements once you've told so that your confidant is clear about whom they can share the information with. Another DI parent, who understands these issues and who doesn't overlap with your daily life, may be a wonderful choice, respectful of the sacredness of this confidence.

If you have an indiscreet relative or friend, you may face a very difficult judgment call about how open to be with him or her. A gossipy, actively alcoholic, or otherwise uncontrolled relative can expand your inner circle to include unintended "confidants," and you certainly don't want your child to hear a drunken, bizarre, or critical interpretation of his conception. You could go "wide open," so that everyone hears of DI from you, including your child at a very young age. You could explain to other confidants why you haven't confided in this person, asking them to honor your decision. Or you may choose to tell no one, or no one close to this indiscreet relative or friend, until your child understands DI.

HOW DO YOU DECIDE TO GO AHEAD WITH DONOR INSEMINATION?

Determining whether or not DI is right for you will be a unique process for each person. For couples it must also be a joint decision and is well worth hashing over from many different perspectives. Any losses that brought you to DI, including the loss of your biological "dream child," need to be grieved and accepted. Jean writes:

> Dr. Cooper wisely suggested I put on the brakes and consider the grieving process for what we'd not be able to do—have a child genetically related to us. She asked a simple question: what would I miss most about not having a child that was related to Josh. I started to answer and lost it. I spent most of the rest of the hour talking through floods of tears. Dr. Cooper recommended we talk to a counselor and gave us two to consider. We were both a bit tentative about this, as we didn't object in principle but had never been to see a counselor. We agreed that we'd go to one meeting, and if we didn't think things clicked, we'd just not go again. We ended up seeing Carol almost every week for about six months.

Some people struggle with very negative reactions to DI. As a RESOLVE member writes:

> At first I could not even consider this as a possibility. After all, how could I watch my wife carry another man's child and be constantly reminded of my own ineptness? I was also torn by guilt for denying my wife the opportunity to experience a pregnancy. I often wished that this option did not even exist, so that I would not have to deal with these feelings.[22]

The time needed to work through these issues is longer for some than for others.[23] A quick decision could lead to missteps, overlooking asking a brother to be the donor, or avoiding the reality that the relationship would fare better if children arrived via adoption.

Coming to Agreement with Your Spouse

If only one of you feels comfortable with DI, it may seem like you'll never be able to get together on this. Some couples end up in opposing camps, one arguing pro and the other con. As Linda Hunt Anton explains in *Never to Be a Mother*:

When we humans invest emotionally in a decision, a plan, an idea, we tend to close our minds to sound, persuasive arguments that support . . . the positive aspects of the side the other person champions. . . . Both alternatives have merit; both have drawbacks.[24]

Laura Alper also looks at communication breakdowns during times of conflict.

A common experience is, during one of those conflict-ridden moments when your partner seems to hammer you with his or her bias, you may find your body digging in its proverbial heels . . . prepared to defend your beliefs and beat down opposition. This usually results in what I call "ping-pong match"—a rapid-fire interchange characterized by very little listening or understanding . . . which can result in hurt feelings, frustration, threats, anger, discord, misunderstanding and misery. . . . Commit yourself to learning about your partner's viewpoints. . . . You can listen to an opposing view without joining it.[25]

Anger is often a cover for grief and anxiety. Some couples have no conflict. Alison writes that after a failed vasectomy reversal led to DI, "My husband was wonderful. Though he never wanted to have more children—he's fifty-three, with a son twenty-five—he realized how important it was to me and decided that it was more important for me to have a child than it was for him not to." Lisa and Eric explain their views in *In Pursuit of Pregnancy*:

LISA: I always wanted to be a parent with Eric. I decided that it didn't matter a bit whether we adopted, used a donor, or had our own. Eric convinced me to try AID first. . . .

ERIC: My feeling was that I wasn't going to be cheated again . . . out of going through a pregnancy with Lisa.[26]

Becki writes of Steve waiting for her to decide.

He wants a child to love—he isn't concerned with how we accomplish that. . . . We have had a very hard time talking about this issue because we try so hard not to hurt each other. . . . But when we did talk about it, it only took him a couple of days to think before he was ready to try it. It had taken me much longer—I had to reconcile myself to the fact that Steve and I probably will never have a biological child.

What approaches might help you decide? Start a list of all the upsetting thoughts, feelings, concerns, and images that arise when you think of DI. Looking at these negatives may be painful, but if you can image how you might overcome or cope in the face of these possibilities, you may have the courage to proceed. Very often this type of exercise gets labeled as negative thinking. You are not saying these things will happen—your worst fears couldn't possibly ALL happen. Nan writes:

> George actually felt more comfortable with DI than I, feeling it made more sense since we had the maternal history and control over the pre-natal care. To me, there was something weird about "adopting" (to use the word of George's urologist) sperm. Not only whose, but what kind of baby would I have?

Elizabeth was more concerned with her husband's feelings. "He didn't like the idea of my being treated with another man's sperm, partially because his ex-wife had an affair." In a powerful article, Tom lists his major concerns:

> First, the threat that I would be excluded in some way from the process of our having children. Second, that the child would somehow seem more Joanna's than mine, both to us and to my side of the extended family. Third, that the donor would somehow look over our lives and be present in our family as a rival. Fourth, that these factors would creep in and damage our marriage.[27]

Once you've made such a list, you can then examine each concern. Many will seem less ominous when brought out in the open.[28] Tom tackles the negative assumptions:

A rival? Some green-horn who had masturbated in a beaker was supposed to be my baby-making rival after Joanna and I spent so many months discussing and carrying out this deeply consuming, deeply spiritual and deeply physical process together. At this point in our effort, the idea was laughable to me.[29]

You might fear an item on your list is irreconcilable, so threatening to your sense of self or your relationship that you doubt you'll be able to proceed with DI. This may again get you in touch with all the pain that first hit when you learned of the diagnosis that would bring you to DI. A man who thought he had accepted infertility may again feel very inadequate comparing himself to a "super-fertile" donor. Sometimes these feelings can be worked through, and at other times couples come to the conclusion they shouldn't proceed.

You can also make a list of the pros. Kristi writes, "I wanted to have control of the nutrition that went into this child. And I wanted to nurse, to feel bonded . . . right away, in the womb. I wanted the best for my child." Chris discovered John had a "more analytical view of things and had chosen DI over adoption because we could then at least achieve a 50 percent genetically related kid!" DI offers the hope of fairly quickly becoming parents, of having a newborn. For some people it also offers the relief of not passing on family genes that aren't so great. As Ben puts it, "If you knew some of my relatives, you'd understand why part of me even felt DI was preferable." For those with clearly transmittable conditions, the advantages of a fresh genetic start are unmistakable.

Many people assume that listing the pros and cons will make the decision obvious—you go with the longer list. In fact, just one glaring item pro or con can tip the scales. For some, a list confirms that the decision is tough to make, with equally compelling arguments for and against DI. And there will never be a 100 percent decision at this point (although you will read of parents who are so happy that they now feel 100 percent certain DI was a miraculous, meant-to-be choice). For now, a majority decision may suffice, as long as you aren't tormented emotionally or maritally by the minority concerns. As Merle Bombardieri states in *The Baby Decision*, "We humans are ambivalent because we're aware of other possibilities, because we know we're giving up one thing to have another."[30] Donna puts it well:

> I was the one who didn't want to do DI; Harry was fine with it. I was grief-stricken that I would not be able to have his baby. When I was finally able to accept this, it worked quickly. Now 99 percent of the time I'm thrilled, but 1 percent of the time I am crushed that I'm not carrying Harry's baby—and that's when I call for a counseling session.

Searching for Information

A well-informed decision is always ideal, so it's very frustrating to find so little information on DI. The research that has been done on DI is reassuring. As psychologist Andrea Braverman concludes:

> In measures of attachment, marital adjustment, and parental feelings, the donor insemination group measured as well or better on all dimensions. . . . Perhaps these families have been overpathologized by the assumption that there has to be a disruption in intrafamilial relations based on genetic differences.[31]

Another study, in *Child Development*, concludes:

> Genetic ties are less important for family functioning than a strong desire for parenthood . . . the suggestion that DI fathers would have difficulty in relating to their children is not supported by the results of this study.[32]

While you are searching for information on DI, you may feel you should also gather information on other options. Many couples use the method of ruling out other alternatives to come to a DI decision. Keep as open a mind as possible in case DI doesn't work. But for some couples DI clearly becomes the "only choice" once they've examined the alternatives of continuing to try for a pregnancy together, adopting, or living without children. While most couples exhaust all hopes for a genetically shared pregnancy, some need to be sure they haven't overlooked any medical options. Adoption is important to consider, especially if a couple can't come to an agreement about DI. One study of DI parents found most had considered adoption. Some couples look at resolving to live without children, accepting child-free living, but this can seem like a 180-degree turn.[33] Any alternative that brings a child quickly looks better than a child-free lifestyle. But for many, it's sad but true that the only child they want is the dream child they now can't have, the baby they would have created together. Nicki struggled with her decision:

> For a few months, we wrestled with the idea of . . . remaining child-free. The thought of becoming a parent was scary enough. I wondered if our situation was God's way of saying that maybe we shouldn't have kids . . . if we were playing God, by going through with DI.

It's important to know you can say no, and you should *at least* say "not yet" if no family-building alternative appeals to you.

If You're Still Undecided

Even if you have worked hard to resolve all the issues you've identified, you may still be stuck. Some couples can't seem to get to yes on DI but don't want to decide no. You may need to make a conscious decision to postpone the decision.[34] This isn't easy, as reminders of your childlessness are everywhere. But time off from decision making may help the reluctant person grieve and gain perspective on DI. A break may help the person who's been nudging toward DI to look at other alternatives. This break is a wise time to attend workshops, seek out counseling, and talk to others who've faced the same decision.

One decision-making deal can be agreeing to look ahead to see how you might, theoretically, do DI. This isn't a promise that you will go ahead with DI; it's just an exploration. You may take a look at sperm bank materials and come across one long profile that's tremendously reassuring. You may explore donor options and realize you'll be able to do DI only with a known donor. You may realize you could do DI without the extended family's ever needing to know about it. You don't have to approve of all DI practices, just see if there's one approach that is acceptable for you.

Perhaps DI itself isn't even the problem. Your indecision may stem more from fear of making a mistake, procrastination, or anger at others' expectations. You may be stuck because your needs always came second, you're afraid to rock the boat, or you feel guilty getting your own way. You may need to be very sure of your relationship before adding DI's challenges.

Seeking Others' Help with Decision Making

If you're continuing to feel unsure about DI, you may need a fresh perspective and some support. Many people are surprised to find they want their parents' approval before beginning. They at least want to know where the family would stand on DI.[35] Leigh remembers:

> We fought for three days straight and then we decided to let our families know what was going on. . . . Peter needed to talk it out with me and his family and friends before he came to the realization that he would like a child who was biologically connected to me.

Sarah and Andy feared her family would be disapproving but needed to talk to them anyway.

> We were more worried about my family because their first grandchild would be conceived in an unusual way. Andy and I sat down with my parents and sister (who knew and was very excited for us) . . . my good Italian Catholic mother left us speechless! They asked questions, which Andy mostly answered, about the procedure, when we were going to start, etc., and my mother was so happy she was going to be a grandmother that the baby could fall out of the sky for all she cares. They opened a bottle of champagne and we all toasted. . . . Our families' support erased doubts for Andy and he's ready to go for it.

Mary's Irish Catholic dad did object by raising potential problems with each alternative. Mary finally blew up and cleared the air.

> "Dad, you don't seem to realize that, for us, creating a family is fraught with all sorts of risks, medical, financial, physical, and emotional. None of our choices, ICSI [intracytoplasmic sperm injection], adoption, or donor insemination, is going to be risk-free. This is the way it is for us!"

While Mary's father did offer his blessing, not all parents can. You may need to turn to your closest sibling or the friend with solid advice in past crises.

Some people also need to seek out pastoral counseling. It's important not to proceed with any option if DI would put you in ethical conflict or alienate you from your faith. Unfortunately, you may already be struggling with faith issues. Many have already survived tragic events and terrible news in seeking to "be fruitful and multiply." If you talk with a clergyperson who knows little about DI, he may only explain official doctrine to you. On the other hand, many pastoral counselors see DI, freely chosen, as a matter of conscience, too complex to be designated as sinful or harmful for all. They can help you discern what Kristi referrs to as "our own personal faith, not the church's belief."

It can also help to talk with an infertility counselor who has helped others through this stage of decision making. If you might hold back with a counselor affiliated with your medical team, then ask for an independent counselor. Unless you get your worries dealt with, *you* may keep yourself from proceeding. Chris remembers, "I was concerned that we had grief issues that were unresolved. I was especially concerned about my husband, as he is the kind of guy who will talk about 'sperm' and not feelings." In hindsight, many DI parents do wish they had sought out counseling specific to DI. In one study of DI parents, 83 percent felt that counseling should be available—but 91 percent hadn't received any.[36]

Talking with DI parents can also bring tremendous relief. Two months after her husband's diagnosis, Nicki was in complete confusion and called their RESOLVE chapter's DI support line.

We spent three hours on the phone with a couple who had been through the exact same thing as us! We met them and their children and we've fallen in love with this family. They gave us a lot of hope and positive feelings. . . . I found myself thinking about their children and how *normal* they looked. No weirdness, no "scarlet DI" pinned to their coats!

If DI Is Not for You

How would you decide DI isn't for you? For some people there is simply another option that is more appealing. For others there is some aspect of DI that they clearly find unacceptable: they don't want anxiety about differences in their relationship with their child; they don't want to deal with societal attitudes toward DI; and so on. Admitting that DI isn't acceptable may bring terrible grief to one or both members of a couple. Lisa's story appeared in *Infertility: The Emotional Journey.*

> More than anything I wish donor sperm could be an option for us, but it isn't an option for Bill. . . . I resent that he will not at this point even consider it, but I also understand and respect his right to his feelings. I think Bill resents that I want donor sperm to be an option.[37]

Not all couples find a way to work this through. The inability to agree on DI may even signal an irreconcilable difference in the relationship. Some couples realize they were never equally committed to parenting and are now very far apart. They don't want to risk parenting conflicts leading to divorce after DI.

Many couples find another pathway to resolution. Jean and Josh's counseling sessions helped them rule out donor insemination. Jean writes of her struggle to accept that only adoption would work for Josh:

> I was convinced for a while that Josh really didn't believe the things he was saying about DI . . . he was raising what I saw to be roadblocks. . . . The sessions with Carol helped me figure out that if I wanted to do this, adoption was the only option where there was a prayer we'd both agree. . . . I wanted Josh to acknowledge the enormity (to me) of what I was giving up by agreeing to drop consideration of DI. . . . I could not be certain

that he'd ever make that kind of sacrifice for me. . . . I think when you
love someone, you have to be willing to accept that there are these
unknowns and proceed anyway, and so I have.

Their shared joy in their son's adoption has helped heal memories of
difficult decision making.

●

When the DI decision is very difficult, forgiveness and patience
become vital. The reluctant person needs to be self-forgiving. Men may
feel guilty that their physical problems ruled out a shared pregnancy
and now their reluctance is delaying or ending hopes for a pregnancy.
It's best if the impatient person can avoid pushing. Some couples need
to limit and structure their time on the topic, choosing other confidants who can help each sort out how to break the stalemate. Keep in
mind the ultimate goal, to make a choice that both of you will be at
peace with, that will strengthen your family ties. Laney writes:

> What stands out, above all else, is the importance of trusting and listen-
> ing to our own feelings, that each of us looked to our own heart and soul
> for guidance. . . . There was no cookbook to follow, and the ingredients,
> combinations, and methods were many. By honoring and respecting our
> own values and intuitions as individuals and as a couple, we started our
> family on very solid ground.

Chapter Three

Understanding Your Donor Options

We didn't know we had any options when we began using donor insemination. Our highly regarded infertility specialist had his own sperm bank, which provided no written information about the donors. I thought this doctor was progressive because he had a counselor with whom all DI couples needed to talk. She chose our donor from a picture of Bob and a few features we requested. I had no reason to doubt his methods or question him about other donor options. He led us to believe he had the best-quality specimens, and we wanted a baby.

So away we went into the world of parenthood, with only a basic medical history for the children we were planning to tell of their origin. I'd love to blame our lack of information only on the doctor's system, but the truth is I'm not sure either of us could've handled it any other way at the time. I was still thinking of the donor as just a vial of sperm and wanted no identifying information, not even the bare facts the doctor was willing to furnish. During my second pregnancy (with the same donor), a couple we met from the RESOLVE donor insemination support group showed me all the information they got from their bank. My thoughts were, "How could they want to know all that?"

With more knowledge and support, maybe we would've chosen a donor differently. But then we wouldn't have our two beautiful children, and that is unthinkable.

—Heidi

H istorically, *options* wasn't a word associated with donor selection, at least not for the parents-to-be. Physicians chose the donor for each cycle, and most practices had a limited number of donors at any one time. Parents of older children may feel some envy of the many options now available. For them donor selection was a matter of trust, not choice.

But you may envy parents who didn't have to choose. It's difficult to navigate this new world of profiles and specimen availability. It's confusing to also have the option of asking someone you know to donate sperm. Some can't proceed, can't even be sure that DI is for them, until they understand every option. You have to choose the approach that allows you to be at peace with your child's genetic heritage and your role in making this choice for her.

Nowadays you can learn a great deal about the donor whose genes may someday be grafted onto your family tree. You may feel confused if the donor's genetic heritage matters a lot to you. After all, couples may feel the need to downplay the role of genes as they face the husband's loss of genetic connection.

If you don't find donor selection terribly distressing, you may be surprised by this chapter. Some view the choice of a donor as relatively unimportant. They emphasize the randomness of genetics and focus on nurture more than nature. Some parents-to-be are so ready to move on that they barely hesitate over donor selection. Some are protecting themselves and acknowledge they'd rather not face too many details. Some fear they would be so obsessive and critical that long profiles would mean long delays. Some come to feel, after a few cycles, that it's just not worth agonizing about. Wendy and Francis chose their first donor carefully and felt great about his profile. Then he wasn't available for the second cycle, and they chose a slightly less perfect match. By the time they were picking their fourth donor, they quipped, "We don't care, just send sperm! Send *any* sperm!"

The History of Donor Selection

In the days of fresh sperm, physicians feared public outrage or legal action—against them, their donors, or the families created with their help. Recent histories of infertility portray a past when insemination even with a husband's sperm was scandalous.[1] The American Fertility Society took some steps to legitimize DI.

> As the practice grew, so did public visibility and controversy. In 1954, another DI child was at the center of a highly publicized divorce case. . . . A Superior Court judge ruled that not only was the child illegitimate, but his mother was guilty of adultery, even though the husband had fully approved the procedure. DI, said the judge, was "contrary to public policy and good morals." . . . In 1955, Dr. Alan Guttmacher . . . concluded that the Society could not remain silent on the issue any longer. . . . [He] introduced his resolution at the . . . 11th Annual Meeting. . . . The ensuing discussion may have been the lengthiest in the Society's history. . . . News of the resolution was carried in . . . the media, but its biggest effect was to prompt human-interest stories in various magazines . . . humanizing the technique and probably making it more acceptable to the public at large.[2]

To ensure the protection of donors, protocols went beyond anonymity.[3] Often more than one donor was used per cycle to deliberately confuse paternity (in a time before DNA testing offered a conclusive paternity test). Records were destroyed. Physicians made promises of lifelong protection from any contact, as if secrecy were of paramount importance to all parties. Physicians protectively kept DI from public view.

The scene began to change when it became possible to freeze sperm. In 1953 *Nature* reported on the first baby conceived with frozen sperm.[4] Once sperm banks could ship frozen specimens nationwide, donor recruitment was no longer a private relationship between a medical practice and its local donors.

In the 1980s DI continued to draw mixed public reactions—when the topic was raised at all. Donor recruitment got particularly negative attention when linked with eugenics. The "science" of eugenics, which focused on improving the gene pool,[5] became associated with Hitler's plan for a "master race." The Repository of Germinal Choice, also referred to as the "Genius Bank" or the "Nobel Prize Bank," drew media attention.

> Back in 1980, when millionaire Robert Graham founded the Repository for Germinal Choice, in Escondido, Calif., he was dead serious about improving the human race. Graham proudly announced that he had collected the semen of three Nobel laureates, and other superior intellects, in order to sire children who would rise above, as Graham once wrote, the "huge masses of those with ordinary minds." Today, Graham, 84, and his enterprise are still going strong. . . . Graham is equally picky about the women who want to buy his bank's sperm. "We'll drop women who are really disappointing," he says. "There's no use wasting the best sperm on an inferior person."[6]

Although some clients of Graham's bank did have an interest in eugenics, others worried about the sperm quality of accomplished but older donors.[7] Most patients shared with their doctors a less grandiose goal, finding well-rounded, healthy, fertile donors, not perfect or superior specimens. Most parents-to-be simply wanted to match their family's talents enough so that a child would fit in.

Most doctors wanted to get to know their donors; they continued to recruit local donors and use fresh sperm into the late 1980s. Many used fresh sperm because it worked more quickly, although there were drawbacks, as Chris recounts:

> Could you trust your donor to stay close by if it was a holiday? What if I ovulated on a weekend? And just whom would we be sharing this potential pregnancy with? We had no pictures, no biographies, nothing, just a vague promise that he'd look like John—whatever that meant.

In the fresh sperm days, couples might wait months while their doctor tried to recruit someone fitting that couple's characteristics. The tradition of physicians providing so little information about donors may have developed in part because couples would have been distressed to learn how little "matching" was possible.

The major push toward sperm banks came with AIDS. Before HIV a few sperm banks existed, focusing on self-banking for men undergoing vasectomies or chemotherapy. Some physicians began freezing their donors' sperm for convenience, for times when a donor couldn't provide fresh sperm at ovulation. The cost of cryobanking equipment and personnel was significant, feasible only at large medical centers. But then the risks of HIV transmission came to be understood.[8] In 1988 the American Fertility Society, the professional organization for infertility specialists, recommended that fresh sperm no longer be used and that frozen specimens be quarantined for six months, until the donor could be retested and found negative for HIV antibodies.[9]

Regulation of DI has increased as an industry of commercial banks, with fiscal pressures and organizational policies, has evolved. A number of professional organizations issue regulatory guidelines for laboratory procedures and donor screening. The Food and Drug Administration (FDA) has found the American Association of Tissue Banks' (AATB) Reproductive Council very thorough in screening for infectious diseases. States, most notably New York, have mandated strict standards to be met before granting licenses to sell specimens. A bank needs to track which accreditation processes are necessary to reassure doctors and recipients. As the cost and complexity of screening a donor become prohibitive for all but the largest banks, small, physician-controlled banks may be forced to consolidate or close.

The screening of donors will continue to expand. Banks often say about one in ten applicants are accepted as donors. Once freezing became standard, many applicants "flunked" because their sperm didn't thaw well. Donors must have a clean bill of health, personally and in their immediate family, and be attractive, personable, and very fertile.

Barbara Raboy, founder of the Sperm Bank of California, explains the rigors of donor screening:

> Donors don't sign a contract until their sixth visit to the sperm bank, after they've been oriented, interrogated, subjected to rectal, throat and urethral swabs, and otherwise palpated and probed. Men hoping to donate sperm complete a twelve-page questionnaire in which they must reveal details about their diet, their penchant for steam rooms, and their exposure to everything from radiation to flea powder. And they must say whether any of their relatives, including cousins, ever suffered from any of a pages-long list of diseases common and obscure. An additional HIV questionnaire presses them for details of their sexual behavior.[10]

New tests for infectious diseases and genetically transmittable conditions continue to emerge.[11] While you may not fully understand the latest in testing, you should ask your bank to document that it meets professional standards.

Sperm Banks' Expanding Options

You have choices among donors and in approaches to picking one. Most banks supply a catalog listing current donors, identifying some characteristics: ethnic origin, hair color and texture, eye color, complexion, blood type, height, weight, occupation, and interests. If the information you need isn't in the catalog—for example, you want a Jewish donor and religion isn't listed—you can call the bank for help.

Once you've identified one or more donors of interest, banks can help you pick among these tentative choices. Most have summary forms on each donor, often referred to as "short profiles." Usually a few are provided free of charge or for a nominal fee if you want to learn more about a large number of donors. California Cryobank was the first bank to allow Internet downloading. Many banks also offer "long profiles" that give a better sense of the donor by outlining his academic history, talents, motivations, or family background. California Cryobank's long profile, for example, asks the donor to rate his relatives' personalities and list their occupations, a reminder that you're not picking just a young man but also his family's "gene pool." Some parents-to-be are looking carefully at long profiles because someday their grown child will read his donor's. Because the fees for long profiles can add up (each bank sets its own fee, and ten dollars each isn't unusual), use these as a final check on the small group of donors you've narrowed down. Sometimes one piece of information can capture your attention. For one couple the clincher in their choice of a donor was the donor's mom, a former ballerina.

Banks try out creative approaches to donor selection. Some may not stand the test of time, while others may later be seen as innovations in the field and be adopted by other banks. An early innovation was asking donors to write about themselves. Even brief answers to questions about motivation or personality can provide some reassurance to a parent-to-be now or an adult child later. Biogenetics developed questions about the donor's lifestyle. Xytex asked donors to write autobiographical essays. California Cryobank guided donors through audiotaped conversations. Innovations in accessing donor information will also continue to develop. Cryogenic Laboratories first developed computerized matching, which it calls DADS—Data Assisted Donor Selection. The initial idea was for doctors to set up an in-office terminal so that patients considering DI could input what they were looking for in a donor and get a printout of profiles on current donors who fit these criteria. Some banks, such as Fairfax Cryobank, have set up Web sites, which offer the advantage of learning about donor options from the privacy of home.

For recipients interested in more in-depth matching on a donor's appearance, some banks have a service usually referred to as photo matching. A staff person will compare any pictures you provide to the pictures on file of each donor you've pre-selected, with an hourly charge for this sometimes time-consuming process. Xytex took the next step, offering photographs of the donor as an adult or as a child, accompanied by the donor's essay and long profile. This service obviously requires the donor's consent, because a photo along with information about his life might increase the chances of his being identified, for example, by an adult child later searching college yearbooks.

One of the most controversial sperm bank approaches has been guaranteeing the release of the donor's identity to DI children at the age of majority. This protects the rights of the child, who wasn't able to consent to anonymous DI. The Sperm Bank of California was the first to offer an identity-release program, in 1983, soon after its opening, and for many years was the only bank allowing this option. Because one column in its catalog of donors indicates a "yes" or "no" decision by the donor about permission to release his identity to a child over eighteen, these "open" donors are often referred to as "yes" donors. The program proved so popular that the small bank couldn't begin to keep up with the nationwide demand for its identity-release donors. Other banks are beginning to develop similar guaranteed identity-release options, but this approach hasn't been supported by AATB guidelines, which reflect a tradition of anonymity so strong that it's presumed to be vital to DI practice.

A differing approach has been taken by banks like California Cryobank, which refers to its plans for responding to requests as an "openness policy." These banks commit to trying to contact the donor with any requests from those conceived with his sperm, once they've reached adulthood. But the option of responding to any requests will remain with the donor. The guiding belief is that no donor should be allowed to make a permanent decision about whether to release or not release. Banks will forward requests to the donor as the years go by and hope that he'll consider each, but they won't lock him in early on.

Any approach assumes that the bank or the adult child will be able to locate the donor years in the future. This is possible using the donor's social security number; for the small cost of a credit check, the bank can find a current address for almost anyone. What may be more difficult to find are support services for donors, adult children, or parents to help them make decisions about how to move from anonymity toward greater openness and to get the most out of any form of contact.

Some banks are rapidly changing. Not long after adding long profiles, the New England Cryobank began to ask donor applicants about their willingness to have contact, either with a recipient now or with a child over eighteen. We've gone from no profiles to identity release in a very brief time.

The expectations of recipients have driven the industry to become consumer responsive. In 1995 Fairfax Cryobank announced that it would provide personal profiles that were longer than its earlier forms, which were essentially short profiles. When asked how that decision was reached, the bank acknowledged that consumer demand had necessitated the policy change. Above and beyond written information, banks provide customer-service staff who can sometimes ease fears and clarify information about bank policies or about a specific donor's profile. Some services are obviously costly for a bank to provide, such as California Cryobank's decision to make the geneticist on staff available to answer questions or provide counseling.

Some professionals believe these services have gone too far. As Dr. Gabor Huszar, an andrologist at the Yale University School of Medicine, put it, "When couples see these menus of donors they start believing that if they want a left-handed Albanian baby who grows up to play baseball, like music, and develop a taste for stuffed cabbage, they can get one."[12] Human genetics is never so simple, nor the inheritance of traits so predictable. Nevertheless, many parents-to-be have welcomed the added access to information, even if it might not correlate at all with scientifically proven factors in genetic transmission. Some find it easier to go ahead with inseminations if the donor seems less a stranger. Some feel more prepared to tell their child, while others, unsure of telling, assume they'll be more at peace with letting a positive memory of the donor fade over time.

Some concerns in sperm banking deserve further analysis. One is the cost and adequacy of specimens. Banks must set per-vial and shipping charges high enough to cover all operational costs: customer-service and scientific personnel, processing and freezing equipment, screening tests, and so on. You're paying for every cost—there are no federal, state, or nonprofit funds underwriting sperm bank services. Between four and ten vials can result from one "donation," but researchers still debate ideal standards.[13]

There are also questions about documenting the number of pregnancies achieved with each donor's sperm. Many parents don't report pregnancies to sperm banks, to protect their privacy. Banks will only "retire" a donor if they've been notified of his maximum number of births. If a donor continues to be used, this increases the small but terrifying risk that two half-siblings, unaware of DI origins, might reproduce—a greater worry in fresh sperm days when doctors used local donors to create local families. Now that sperm is shipped all over the country, limits such as ten live births are less important than distributing specimens from any given donor over many states. But banks need recipients' help to track pregnancies.

Who Are the Sperm Bank Donors?

Some of the anxiety many couples have about DI centers around their inability to learn much about sperm donors. Who are these men, why are they doing this, and where do they come from? Secrecy makes that information difficult to come by. Donors and sperm banks haven't had a very positive reputation. Negative stereotypes must change if DI is to become an accepted, nonstigmatized family-building alternative. Society is becoming more comfortable with masturbation as a normal activity, so maybe its role in DI will draw less ridicule. Possibly policies against openness must change before donors can be viewed as honest and altruistic.

While most donors are in their early twenties, the image of the single, childless student fits only a percentage of donors. Banks advertise at universities because students are most likely intelligent, and the flexibility of scheduling donating around academic work is very appealing to students. Banks affiliated with medical centers still have a sizable percentage of donors in the medical field, but donors are recruited from all walks of life. They're selected for intelligence, health, attractiveness, and positive personality traits—though it's wise to remember that these factors are subject to a degree of interpretation by staff members who meet several times with the applicants. Donors are paid a fee of thirty-five to fifty dollars for an ejaculate of adequate quality, which requires some abstinence before each visit to the bank.

There's a movement toward unpaid donation only. This is partly to remove even the small financial incentive to conceal damaging information. But it is also to remove any image of donors involved in a commercial exchange and to prevent childrens' feeling bad about resulting from this. The FDA would like all sperm and egg donors to be unpaid, as other tissue donors are. The fear among professionals and parents-to-be is that there would be a dramatic increase in the wait for specimens or far less choice in donors.

It may be that increasing the social acceptability of DI would bring in many new men to donate. Most people assume that men donate sperm exclusively for the financial compensation. Ken Daniels, a researcher in New Zealand, has written on the implications of shifting from "marketed" sperm to "gifted" sperm.[14] He found that the most common motivation for a small sample of donors was helping infertile couples; over half said they'd still donate if there was no payment or reimbursement of expenses.[15] Of course, some donors do have a strong financial motivation. As one donor writes:

> I was unsure how my friends and fiancee would react, and I was also uneasy about how awkward the actual process of becoming a donor would be. . . .
> To be totally honest, I overcame my reservations simply because I needed the money. Med school has a tendency to put you in the poor house.

A property manager with two kids, interviewed in a 1992 article, donated so he could afford to spend more time with his children and still pay for their college later. But money wasn't his only motivation, as he explains:

> I work with a guy whose wife is having trouble conceiving, and I see the trouble and frustration they go through. It made me feel kind of good that I could help some of these people. On the other hand, I say to myself, "What if I create a child who's born into a really bad situation?" But I put the burden of finding the right people on the sperm bank. I let them worry about the matchmaking, so to speak.[16]

This donor demonstrates that many men are fully aware of and concerned about the controversies regarding third-party reproduction. A donor in medical school writes of many such concerns in his essay:

> My only thoughts and feelings about the children that I have helped produce are that I hope that they are healthy and that I hope the parents are deserving and know how to love the child and be good parents. I do not feel that the child is mine or that I should have the right to meet him/her later, nor do I feel that I have done anything immoral or wrong. . . . I would have no problem at all submitting a photo or even giving an interview to the potential recipients. . . . If I later found that I had a genetic illness, I would definitely tell the bank and end my days of donation.

Ken Daniels represents a growing number of professionals concerned that donors are being treated as vendors, with little concern for long-term impact on them.[17] The vast majority of donors he interviewed reported wanting to know the outcome of their donation, and thinking about the children conceived.[18]

A donor's altruistic concern and empathy can be for the parents-to-be as well as for the children. As a married donor in a Cryogenic Laboratories videotape puts it, "Our kids are so wonderful, we could help other people have that same happiness we have." In 1991 two therapists specializing in infertility counseling, Patricia Mahlstedt and Kris Probasco, published research on donors' attitudes. They gathered donors' messages to children:

"I want you to know that the small part I played in your creation has made me very proud, and I wish you all the best your life has to offer."

"Be aware of the small sacrifices that your parents have made on your behalf. Artificial insemination is a difficult choice, and to have made it means your parents considered having you to be worth the struggle."

"I am glad I could help in your conception but your real parents are the ones who raised you and took care of you. I hope you find life beautiful. Be happy!"[19]

David, interviewed for an article by DI mom Tamar Abrams, donated to learn more about his genetic history; he saw the fee as payment for his time. "I get to provide a gift for couples and single women."[20] Patrick and Emily chose their donor because he was motivated by infertility in his immediate family. "We felt that he'd experienced the pain and frustration of a loved one, possibly a sister." However, you'll find quite a range of donor motivations. One reporter found a profile of someone less focused on helping. "I believe I am genetically superior to most people," writes California Cryobank's Number 143. "I seem to excel at everything I attempt. I have an IQ of 127."[21]

The donor's honesty and accuracy are often a concern. If money is the incentive to donate, many couples ask themselves what keeps donors from lying. The anonymous author of "Confessions of a Sperm Donor" reveals:

> There was a section on substance abuse: Had I ever tried pot? . . . Here I admit to fudging a little. . . . I was reluctant to put on paper the full extent of my former use . . . my deception does point up a serious issue. If, for example, my family had a history of mental retardation and I chose to keep it a secret, it would have been difficult for the sperm bank to find out.[22]

David "was 100-percent honest on my donor history. . . . I called all my relatives to get their histories, and I told them what I was doing."[23]

Many wish that his approach would become the norm, since a good percentage of young men haven't yet learned about all their relatives' illnesses, especially stigmatizing conditions like depression. If a donor knows such information, he certainly would be asked to reveal it. The application process is lengthy, with checks and cross-checks, so he can't casually overlook anything important. And donors are read the riot act, told they'll share in any legal liability, as well as obvious ethical culpability, if they conceal anything.

Another major area of concern is donor motivation to meet the needs of grown children, many of whom will someday know of their donor conception. Banks and doctors fear that potential donors would be scared off by the possibility of future meetings. Certainly a structured way to meet any requests from adult children would be much more appealing to a donor than having a twenty-something stranger knocking on his door unannounced. As David puts it:

> I am a genetic parent. I have no emotional ties. . . . I would be willing to be contacted by a donor child if he or she went through the sperm bank first. . . . I would love to see photos of the children I've fathered. I would even love to meet the parents.[24]

It will become important for banks to educate donors that contact with young adults could be interesting and to offer options for communication, easing concerns a donor might have.

Most donors are aware of children's needs, however uncomfortable it might be to contemplate meeting them. Mahlstedt and Probasco's research found that almost all donors are willing to provide nonidentifying psychosocial and medical information. They concluded donors are less self-protective and more concerned about recipient families than professionals once thought.[25]

When there's still controversy over anonymously providing background information, it's admirable that a small but growing percentage of donors are willing to release their identity. One donor explains:

I have a friend who's adopted. When I mentioned I was an anonymous donor, she told me in no uncertain terms how much she wished she knew who her biological parents were. That's a very different situation, but I'd like the kid to be able to meet me, if she wants to.[26]

Frank, an identity-release, or "yes" donor at the Sperm Bank of California, has expressed his interest in a meeting someday:

Frank told me he is full of anticipation about that "knock on the door" looming in his future, like a "surprise package eighteen years from now." He envisions a friendship with these children, and admits having to chase away thoughts of how they look, what kind of people they are. "I hope they like me," he adds. About one thing he's fairly certain: they will get in touch with him. "I would. And if they're anything like me, they will too."[27]

The anonymous author of "Confessions of a Sperm Donor" would not volunteer.

I may have given the sperm, but I'd like to think that whoever raised the child would be the real parents. And, to be blunt, I doubt I'd feel any real tie to a child I'd never seen, one that I had helped produce by masturbating into a cup.[28]

Donors interviewed by Mahlstedt and Probasco[29] and by Daniels[30] found a range of reactions, with a sizable percentage willing to meet adult children but others against it.

Many people wonder why banks fear voluntary, mutual-consent open-identity policies when offering this option doesn't seem to be a problem with most donors and recipients. Becki writes:

I'd like it if the program at least made it possible for the donor and the family to make contact in the future, if and when both sides indicate an interest. But our university's program is very opposed to that. In fact, when I talked to one official about this possibility, he said most recipients never even tell the child about the DI procedure.

This distrust of openness may change over time as more families successfully negotiate more open forms of third-party reproduction.

DRAWBACKS TO DELEGATING DONOR DECISIONS

Suggesting that you select a donor represents a radical change from DI tradition. Some doctors remain unconvinced that couples can deal with this reality of DI. When Ellen and Kirk's doctor selected the donor for them, he fully believed this was only proper.

> He explained that he felt it wasn't "healthy" for the recipients to become overly attached to the donor, but if a pregnancy did occur, the donor ID number would be released to us and we could get basic medical and descriptive information. We accepted this as the "normal process." At the time I knew no one else who'd been through this, and it wasn't something you could find information about in your local bookshop.

Similarly, Steve and Becki wanted more information but were put off.

> We were very disappointed in the sketchy information available about the donors. All we received was a list of about ten case numbers with the following information: height and weight; eye, hair, and skin color; ethnic background; occupation and interests (which, in every case, was "sports"). . . . We're very concerned that we won't receive a detailed medical history, although we've been assured that if we need that information in the future, it will be made available. . . . Is this bank thinking in the dark ages or is this the general attitude?

It may be even more frustrating nowadays to hear that such information is sometimes available but not have your requests accepted.

Many doctors require patients considering DI to meet with a staff person to specify the characteristics that are important to them (hair color, eye color, blood type, religion, and such), and then that staff person selects the donor. In fact, some practices explain they want to have permission to order any one of several donors who "match" the husband's (or wife's) physical characteristics, so that if the most closely matched donor isn't available, they'll go to the next best and you won't have to skip a cycle. (The other way to avoid this is to buy and reserve specimens of your first choice, as we'll discuss later.) If you want to do the selection yourself, in some practices you'll actually have to get the doctor's permission. Elizabeth wanted to choose her own donor, but her doctor was against it.

> I didn't feel I was offered much input or any options. My doctor picked out the donor. When I told him I wanted to choose my own, he first only let me see the physical characteristics sheets. His nurse was the one who felt I should be able to see the full sheets and gave me the phone number of the lab person who screened the donors.

Some people prefer to delegate donor selection to the medical team. But no staff person can possibly care as much about your donor's selection as you do. Unless the staff people who deal with sperm bank ordering know patients very well, they'll have little or no idea about your specific preferences. Some people mistakenly presume that their doctor or nurse, who has come to know them after months of infertility treatment, will spend hours choosing, but this is almost never the case. They're extremely busy and often limit their input to medical or genetic inheritance questions. They're also more likely than you to mistakenly overlook one of your preferences, easy to do when juggling orders. You would never forget that you want only an Irish donor or one whose parents both had brown eyes, but a staff person hurrying to fill out orders might. Diana writes of the outcome of delegating donor selection.

> Our clinic picked the donor for patients, supposedly based on the husband's physical characteristics. Some months after our son was born, I decided to get as much information about our donor as the clinic and sperm bank would allow. We had done a lot of reading on the importance of openness, trust, and honesty with adopted children and planned on using this same approach with our son. As it turned out, the records

showed our son's donor was medium height and build, with light hair and hazel eyes. My husband is six foot two, wears an extra-large, and has dark brown hair and brown eyes. (I too, have dark hair and dark eyes.) The technician's "good match" consisted of like blood types. Our son has blond-brown hair and huge blue eyes. But with the irony these situations often seem to engender, our adopted daughter has light brown hair and blue eyes as well. People may ask, "Where did they get the blue eyes?" but they never question the kids' assumed biological connection to each other.

Certainly parents fall in love with their long-awaited child and feel as if he was always meant to be theirs. But most would prefer to be spared any surprises.

Picking a donor may be complicated enough that it takes a team effort, and you'll need to sort out who will cover what base. For you and your child, this "order" has lifelong implications, and you don't want to realize later that disturbing information exists on file, overlooked by your doctor, who was trying to spare you from stress in selecting a donor. Since that information will be available to your child too and its negativity may make you afraid to disclose DI if you'd planned to do so, the avoidance of donor information now can inadvertently make DI more difficult over your lifetime.

Katie and Arthur almost followed the urging of their doctor's assistant, who usually did the donor selection and ordering, to get started with a donor who seemed just fine based on the short profile. They decided to ignore their impatience and wait for the long profile. That showed a history of mild depression and antidepressant treatment, which wouldn't concern many, but given a strong pattern in Katie's family, it made this donor an unwise choice for them. Moreover, Arthur worked in law enforcement, and the donor's recreational drug use bothered him. He was trying to be realistic and not rule out too many donors, because many were honest in mentioning some marijuana use in their long profiles. But with this donor turning to both recreational and prescription drugs, Arthur and Katie felt he was the wrong choice for them. "My kid is going to grow up hanging out with cops, and he might think the donor is a sleazeball even if I don't!"

There are many anxieties about choosing a donor that can lead couples to pull back from this task. Some fear they'll become overwhelmed, unable to make a choice. Some fear details will make the donor all too real at a time when they want some distance. Some feel they shouldn't question this anonymous "gift." Anne remembers her reaction to long profiles: "I recall sitting by the pool at home reading . . . and wondering if we had in fact gone too far. These men were the age of Clyde's oldest biological son. Was I sick?"

Richie had a number of concerns: that his wife would become obsessed with donor selection and delay their getting started, that he'd be jealous of her interest, and that selecting a donor would make him feel like he was "playing God." They worked hard to clarify what they wanted in a donor, delegated someone close to them to search through profiles, and were relieved to hear that one donor was a "perfect match." This compromise of delegating the task to someone who knows you well still requires in-depth examination of what you feel comfortable with, but may be less frustrating and disturbing than spending days surrounded by profiles, especially if you know that one or both of you tends to procrastinate or become obsessed and distracted by minor details. Obviously, intermediaries need to come back to couples if the task isn't clear or if they can only narrow down the choices but feel the final selection must be the couple's. Many counselors would be concerned that an inability to pick the donor reflects unreadiness to live with DI's realities, so do think about what it would take to make donor selection a manageable step toward beginning your family.

SETTING YOUR PRIORITIES

The process of choosing a donor begins with a clarification of your priorities. Your donor search may then become simplified because only certain banks can meet your needs or only one or two donors will be good "matches." One recommendation is to keep notes on your selection process so that you can look back at why you chose as you did. This may be helpful to you in someday talking to your child too.

It can also help to remember that there's no one perfect way to choose a donor. You, and perhaps someday your child, need to know you did the best you could. Choosing a donor is obviously important, but your child's future will be shaped as much by your love and nurture as by her genes. Let's look at some of the priorities important to people, some of the possible approaches to this very difficult task.

Selecting on Genetically Transmittable Characteristics

Physical characteristics are very important to families who aren't certain when or if they'll disclose DI to their child. This was assumed to be the case when catalog formats were first developed in the sperm-banking industry, which is why eye color, hair color and texture, height, and blood type are listed so prominently. The genetics of these traits is quite a bit more complex than the general public's perception. For instance, many people think that two brown-eyed parents will have brown-eyed children, when often both parents have a recessive blue gene. But you probably do need to go with what the general public perceives to be patterns of inheritance. Even if brown-eyed parents can have a blue-eyed baby, you may want to stick to brown-eyed donors so that your children will be more likely to have brown eyes. Stupid questions about differences can become intrusive, especially as your child becomes old enough to wonder why others are asking them. Even a child who knows of DI might resent being singled out as different from others in the family.

When narrowing down the list of donors, many people who wish to be discreet about DI feel that they must select only the husband's characteristics. Others match to the mom-to-be, feeling a double dose of her characteristics will be fine too. The goal in this approach to donor selection is to have the child's characteristics be consistent with the inheritance patterns that could have come from a genetically shared pregnancy. Hair texture, which is listed in catalogs, has a complex inheritance pattern: two straight-haired parents will usually have straight-haired children, two curlies generally have curlies, and a curly and a straight have mostly wavies. This isn't well known, so you might compromise on this more easily than on eye color. Height is more complicated and therefore explainable; it's commonly understood that two short parents can sometimes have tall children, and vice versa. And here's one trait for which a dad often deliberately picks someone dissimilar—if he has always wished to be taller and feels he'd like his child to have that chance. Hair color is the trait frequently joked about with Carol because she has the red hair that couples fear when they ask, "What will we say if a redhead pops out?" This is an example of needing a calm response to any comments when a baby is born. Loved ones aren't asking, "Did red hair show up because you got pregnant with someone else's sperm?" Most people accept any plausible explanation of traits in a child by hearing they've been passed on from any relative, however distant, in either the husband's or the wife's family. You can practice just quietly beaming with pride until you can develop that explanation.

You don't want to drive yourself crazy working out the genetics of each trait. For complex traits, including hair color, height, and skin shade, you may simply want to match as many of these traits as possible to the dad-to-be, just to maximize the chances that your child won't have to deal with odd comments or feel that he doesn't fit in. It can also help to remember that few children look exactly like their parents.

One exception is blood type. While some differences in characteristics can easily be explained away, blood type is best carefully matched if you want to have the option of not telling your child as a preteen about his DI origins. You must choose a donor with a blood type that will give the child a type consistent with one of the wife and husband's possible combinations. You don't want your child to learn in biology class that something isn't right. The Blood Type Table on page 73 shows all the possible donor blood types without going back to the grandparents' types. Check the column of the wife's blood type and the row of the husband's. Where they intersect you'll find the donor blood types you can use.

The same is true with Rh factor, another component of blood type. There's only one "impossibility": no two Rh-negative parents can have an Rh-positive baby, so if both parents are Rh–, the donor must also be Rh–. For medical reasons, even if just the mother is Rh–, the cautious medical advice is to choose a negative donor, because having a second Rh+ fetus developing in a mother who's Rh– can sometimes result in serious anemia for the baby. Unfortunately, Rh– donors are rare, as this trait is present in only 10 percent of the population. So if the wife is Rh– and you want to use an Rh+ donor, check with your doctor, who will educate you about options to protect your pregnancy.

Tobin and Beth found themselves with competing priorities, but the goal to have a healthy pregnancy and baby took precedence. Beth had already had pregnancy losses with an Rh+ donor and was advised to shift to an Rh– donor. But the couple was committed to working only with an identity-release donor, which at that time narrowed their choice down to the Sperm Bank of California's approximately ten identity-release donors. Only one was Rh–, and he was of a very different nationality and appearance than Tobin. They decided they'd let go of the benefits of having their family look alike in order to go into their next round of trying with a good chance for a healthy pregnancy and with a donor who would later meet their child's needs for future information.

Blood Type Table

Find the box where the wife's blood type column and the husband's blood type row intersect. That box lists possible donor blood types that allow the child's blood type to be consistent with the parents'.

NOTE: This table goes back only one generation; a family tree examining the grandparents' blood types might identify a type as implausible.

Wife's Blood Type					
		A	B	AB	O
Husband's Blood Type	A	A, O	any	any	A, O
	B	any	B, O	any	B, O
	AB	AB only	AB only	any	AB
	O	A, O	B, O	O only	O only

Selecting on Appearance

Most couples appreciate services that give them more of a sense of the donor's appearance. Most want their child to "fit" into the family, with similar features and physique, and may feel reassured if the donor looks like the dad-to-be or the mom-to-be. Leigh recalls:

> Gary was adamant about having our children look like me. We weren't going to lie to them and say that they were Gary's children . . . so then why did they have to look like him? . . . As it turned out . . . both children look exactly like me.

Photo matching goes beyond eye and hair color to look at specifics such as the shapes of facial features. In the fresh sperm days, when each doctor recruited a few donors, this level of matching was impossible. You are also unlikely to find it at a small local bank. But if you go to a larger bank with hundreds of donors to choose from, they may offer photo matching. A staff person looks at a set of photos and makes her best estimate of similarities. Ultimately, it's a judgment call based on less than rigorous science, because you can't predict or control what features a child will inherit.

As long as you realize you're only somewhat improving the chances of your child looking like you, you may find it comforting to know you at least tried to select someone similar in appearance. You need to send the bank one or more pictures. It isn't vain to send photos of yourself in your twenties, because that's usually the age of donors to whom you're being matched. If there's a particular facial feature you're looking to match, your deep-set eyes or cleft chin, let the staff person know that. Photo matching provides more reassurance for private parents that they won't be asked where their child got a certain feature.

You may also want to see if you can receive a photo of the donor, the option first offered by Xytex. Because not all donors are comfortable with this, you're immediately reducing your possible choices if you limit yourself to donors with photo files. But some people need to check out resemblances for themselves. More commonly, photos are requested for reassurance that the donor is reasonably attractive, without any odd features.

Selecting on Ethnicity

Some people assume that matching on ethnicity will help them with appearance matching, when in fact there's a wide range of appearances associated with any ethnic group. But ethnicity is also very important for cultural sharing of the dad-to-be's heritage. As one dad puts it, "Being Irish is very important to me, and if my son and I were to travel to Ireland together, I'd want that to be a genuine sharing of heritage, even if our genes originated in different counties of Ireland." Many couples who are unsure when they'll disclose DI to their child feel that matching on ethnicity means giving their child less misinformation because he will indeed belong to his dad's ethnic group.

Some people need to know that the donor shares a similar religious background, a characteristic often linked to ethnic heritage. People who are very involved in their religion may fear that their child could someday be disturbed to learn that the donor didn't share her family's belief system, and could in fact react by feeling this was the cause of any of her own religious conflicts. Sometimes it is wise to look at the long profile before rejecting—or accepting—a donor based on the religion he lists, because only one generation back, his heritage might be quite different.

Selecting on Interests and Talents

Catalogs list occupations and interests, and profiles go into even more depth. Many people need a sense that the donor is "like" them in some way. They at least need to know that the donor isn't terribly dissimilar, and everyone does experience instant aversions as well as attractions. Yet it's important to question to what extent the donor's interests or accomplishments should concern or sway you. Donors are generally young and may have only begun to explore occupations, talents, and interests. His interests are also strongly influenced by what he has been exposed to, which may be fairly limited at his age. However, if the donor says his goal is to become a model, physicist, or doctor and you find his choice personally off-putting, you need to pay attention because you need to feel good about your donor.

On the other hand, curb any tendency you may have toward obsessiveness or perfectionism. Ideally, you will work as a couple to maintain an objective perspective and avoid critical nit-picking. Jim and Shelley laugh together over the donor who was fine in every other way except for listing "baseball card collecting" as a hobby, something Shelley thought was too far outside her realm of acceptable uses of free time.

If you believe this type of information is important, you'd be wise to order long profiles before rejecting donors. With three-generation outlines of such data, you may see a different pattern of family talents. It would be a shame to seek too specifically—for example, for a football player—when the donor came from a family just as athletic as yours but more drawn to soccer or skiing.

Selecting on a Donor's Personal Statements

Some recipients need to have more of a sense of the donor as a person, his values and motivations. It's often assumed this is for the child's sake, to have reassuring material to share later, but it's often as impor-tant to parents-to-be. A woman struggling with the idea of allowing another man's sperm into her body will often feel great relief learning he's a nice guy or caring person.

While some banks have brief answers to personal questions included in their profiles, these questions have always presented some problems. Not all donors are motivated or able to write sensitively. A donor's inclination toward self-disclosure and his talent in expressing himself—or lack thereof—can skew how he comes across. At the point of answering the questions, donors have been through more extensive screening than they ever could have imagined and may simply want to get the process over with. Not fully understanding the purpose of the questions or the impact of their answers on recipients, donors may feel the questions are just more hoops to jump through. It's up to recipi-ents not to become overly alarmed by answers, to interpret them as open-mindedly as possible. When a graduate student answers that he became a donor to cover the cost of books, it's possible to view him as tactless and uncaring of the families he's helping create. His answer could also, however, be interpreted as a sign of honesty, directness, or dedication to his education.

You may well decide to be cautious and pick as positive a profile as you possibly can. This is especially true if you're intending to show the profile to your child twenty years from now and you aren't sure any more access to information will ever become available. After choos-ing two possible donors from the short forms, Maura ordered long profiles.

> One donor's information packet was a joke and not totally unexpected. There wasn't a complete medical history, and the "touchy-feely" ques-tions asked at the end were answered with "I'm doing it for the money." The other donor's information packet revealed someone more like my husband than I would have imagined. This donor also had "great" sperm samples.

If long profiles or other materials exist on potential donors and you're considering someday telling your child of DI, now is the time to look at those. When you're already pregnant, having chosen a donor based on a short profile or having allowed your medical team to choose, it's a bit late to discover something that is distressing given your family's background and values. Get all the information on your chosen donor before you begin so that you know you can accept any minor "flaws" you detect from the profile.

Some banks offer audiotapes and open-ended essays. Listening to a donor's voice, getting a feel for his style in expressing himself, might give you a stronger sense of him. But it might also be confusing; an accent, for example, could make a student here from another country seem even more "foreign" to you. Another drawback is that brief answers, offered without much forethought, can sound pat or simplistic instead of sincere. If videotapes join the options, these will add the distractions of appearance and mannerisms. You may find yourself in a bind, uncertain how much is the right amount of information for you. You may need to trust that any current distress will have plenty of time to fade, to be replaced by reassurance over the years that you pulled out all the stops in selecting the best donor for your family.

Selecting on the Level of Information for Your Child at Adulthood

If you want a guarantee that identifying information will be available to your child someday, your choice of banks will be quickly narrowed. Identity release is rarely promised today, although this may change in years to come. Nonidentifying information, at least of a medical nature, is already considered routine at most banks, and you'll need to decide if this is enough. Maura chose not to use an identity-release bank.

> There were only two labs in California that offered "identified" donors. We felt that we didn't need to get an identified donor if we could get the medical history of the donor and possibly some nonidentifying personal

information. We also felt that access to donor information would change
in the future, like adoption records. We weren't comfortable with using
the identified-donor sperm bank due to its uniqueness and possible over-
use. We decided that we were comfortable giving our child the information that we could obtain at that time.

While some banks are moving slowly toward greater openness, you do
need to think through the implications of working with banks not yet
beginning to address children's requests. One bank, well regarded for
its thorough testing, prides itself on being a "bastion of anonymity."
Some professionals believe that even requesting more contact is a violation of the proper way to cope with DI. Ideally, you'll work with a
bank and medical team committed to at least treating your child's future needs with respect. You'll want compliance with the most flexible standards that have developed to date. For now, that includes a
willingness to hold on to records and to request of the donor that he
later consider requests from anyone conceived with his sperm.

If access to identifying information is vital to you, you'll need to
find which donors have given permission for future release. While the
number of such donors is likely to be small, you may be able to do
somewhat less matching on other characteristics, such as blood type,
because you're planning to tell your child about DI. Jim felt that a
donor's willingness to be identified was almost the only important factor. He wouldn't sacrifice what he believed to be his child's right, even
though that tremendously limited the number of donors he and Shelley
could consider. He was in a DI decision-making group, and the other
members were intrigued. He got some pointed questions, as others
wondered if identity release wasn't a suggestion to the child that searching is vitally important, overemphasizing the donor's role. Other
couples in Jim's group had chosen a bank promising to convey requests
from the child but leaving the option of disclosure up to the donor.
For Jim this wasn't enough. He and Shelley did find an identity-
release donor acceptable to both, but Shelley found the stress of
ordering almost too much.

There's such a high demand for the ID release donors that you're only allowed to order two vials a cycle. You're supposed to call the day of your period and order. I learned quickly that, following these rules, there were never any vials available for the donor of my choice.

This can be particularly difficult if you're planning to have more children and you want to reserve sperm so that they'll be genetically full siblings. Paul, a DI dad, wanted an identity-release donor but admitted being concerned his children might develop unrealistic expectations of their donor, fantasies that wouldn't be fulfilled.

I wouldn't want them to think that they'd be immediately accepted if they suddenly show up at the donor's door and say, "Here I am, Dad!" . . . But I think it would be nice if they did meet him—I'd like to meet him myself. Then . . . whatever works out works out.[31]

NARROWING DOWN YOUR CHOICES

To make a final choice, you'll have to sort out what is most important to you. You may struggle with goals or feelings that seem mutually exclusive—you want to know the donor is attractive but you don't want a photo; you want to preserve your future child's right to information about her genetic heritage but you fear identifying information will send her off searching for a relationship with this man. For couples, the two of you may also want very different things in a donor. If you have strong preferences in many different areas, you may have to search extensively to find even one donor who comes close to a "match." This is why it's common for banks and doctors to provide worksheets asking you to rank what's most important, less important, or totally optional. Some people find it hard to let go of any area, particularly those who worry about later explaining to their adult child why they picked that donor. For others there are only a couple of areas of concern. Matthew and Laurie were especially thorough in selecting their donor.

First, we each made a private list of the ten most important qualities or characteristics we wanted for our donor. We ranked our lists in order from most important to least. Then we shared our lists. There were many similarities but our orders were different. We then chose four of the top cryobanks around the country. Our first scan was for hair and eye color. Funny, that wasn't number one on either list. . . . Second was height and weight. Third, national origin. Then religion. Blood type wasn't important to us since it was our choice to be open with our child and it would have limited our choice a great deal.

These characteristics were available on the initial shortened lists, and the choices helped us narrow down the batch. It was now time to call for the longer donor profiles. We got two to six from each bank. I know that sounds like a lot of work, but this would be our kid so it was worth it; the more we knew about the donor, the better. Now we could evaluate hobbies and grade point averages along with complete health histories. If we were lucky we could dig out bits of personality from donor comments or even handwriting.

It was important for us to stick to the cryobanks and donors that provided more in-depth information since we planned to share this information with our son. . . . The stack was split and we began to read.

We began to chuckle and joke around about what we read and turned a chore into fun. We even started hand signals to describe the habits and characteristics of the donors. One guy wrote he smoked marijuana two times. I'm sure you can guess that hand signal. There were roman noses, wide hands, and vegetarians. At least we could laugh a bit while making one of the hardest decisions of our marriage.

We narrowed the pile down to seven from a combination of banks. Then the calls began. There were all sorts of conventional and creative ways to dig up more information about these donors. Some banks provided a photo-matching service, which we took advantage of. If you're sincere and creative, you can get through to the staff biologist or donor interviewers to delve deeper. When you get these people going, you can squeak out other information, like a feeling about personality or a better indication on what the person looks like. Information like this can be enough to put you over the edge on a certain donor.

Taking charge of the process, as Matthew and Laurie did, can take lots of time, energy, and patience. It's difficult to figure out the protocols for the bank—or banks—you're trying to deal with, your doctor's procedures, and your own needs and constraints. But one group of DI parents came to the consensus that the goal was to think so much about the donor at this stage that you could later let him fade into a vague positive memory of blue eyes or artistic talent or a sweet essay response.

JUST THE FIRST OF MANY DONOR CHOICES?

Nothing seems simple with DI. Once you've become informed about, maybe even comfortable with, donor selection, you realize it will take some effort to keep your donor available. You may be surprised how frequently a donor's supply sells out, at least until the next group of his specimens comes out of quarantine. If you've had a hard time finding an acceptable donor, you may want to make sure you don't have to select another—at least not anytime soon. Grace writes:

> Kind of funny. I thought that when I got married I had chosen the father of my children. Now I got to do it again every couple of cycles. I could never remember from month to month which one we were using . . . "142 isn't available? How about 181? Well, how many do you have? Oh. Well, what about 206? Yeah, two samples please." It was somewhat depersonalizing.

Peggy remembers her frustration after she'd found her perfect donor.

> The woman [on staff at the sperm bank] asked me if I had a second choice. But I never had a second choice because I wanted to decide on the perfect choice for the father of my child and not settle for second best. . . . I practically fell in love with #527 at California Cryobank. I loved his personality. Someone working in the lab told me that he's a great guy. I loved what he wrote about his family. When his sperm was gone I was devastated.

Peggy got caught in a common bind. People often aren't advised how quickly vials on a donor can sell out or how little notice there may be that he's moved out of the area or decided to stop donating. The most effective way to avoid this is to buy lots of vials, but you can pretty quickly max out a credit card limit. Rachel found it worth the cost to avoid "repicking."

> In order to avoid the long and arduous task of choosing a donor every month (often under time constraints), we discovered it was best to buy in bulk (i.e., several vials at a time) and have them stored specifically for us. This meant more of an investment on our part and a different fee schedule, but we found it worth it to avoid some of the mental angst. If we were lucky enough to conceive before our supply was depleted, we decided we'd have the remaining supply stored for our future use and were consoled by the fact that our children might have the same biological connection.

Cheryl, trying on her own, didn't have that option.

> I had a different donor each cycle. Due to financial constraints, I didn't feel that I could afford to "stock up" on sperm that I might not need, and due to demand, the same donor was never available two months in a row.

Matthew and Laurie tried to figure out a way to avoid buying costly amounts of sperm.

> Finally through photo matching we narrowed the list down to two, then picked the closer look-alike. Unfortunately, he was no longer in the program, but we decided to take our chances since 100 samples were available. This information was pried out, since the bank didn't like to disclose that information.

The reason banks don't like to state the number of vials available today is that they could be quickly bought and reserved by tomorrow. For a popular donor, one hundred vials might not be a lot—again, no one realizes how common DI is and how quickly specimens sell.

DECIDING WHETHER TO MOVE
TOWARD A KNOWN DONOR

A very different approach is asking someone you know to donate sperm. One study found that almost half the infertile couples considered asking someone they knew, most often a brother of the husband.[32] For a long time doctors presumed that infertile men felt too threatened or ashamed to consider this option. Some went further, theorizing any need to know the donor was inappropriate.

> It goes without saying that the mother should never know who the donor is, and the donor should certainly not be a member of the husband's family, nor know the identity of the woman. If a man knew who his child is he may attempt to interfere with his upbringing; and all agreed at the Ciba Symposium [physicians' meeting] that this would be disastrous . . . there is no need to tell anyone at all outside the family that the child is not the husband's.[33]

Now doctors have had to reconsider their opinion that families can't cope with known donors. They've seen women donate eggs and carry pregnancies for sisters, friends, even daughters. But there are still those in the medical community who feel it's wrong or worry there's insufficient experience to allow informed consent.

There are many reasons reported for considering known donors: to lower costs, to know more about the donor, to carry on family genes, to avoid being inseminated with a stranger's sperm. Some seek "newly known" donors, recruiting someone according to their own criteria. Amy Blanchard, a psychologist, writes about choosing between known and unknown donors.

> Since the donor is a "real" person, the parents can pass along firsthand information to the child rather than descriptive information from a file. And by far, the greatest advantage is that the offspring and the parents both have access to the donor, and the offspring's "right to know" is maintained.[34]

In *Beyond Infertility,* Susan Cooper, a psychologist, notes, "Some couples who choose known donors do so primarily because they believe that it is unfair to create a child who may suffer from genealogical bewilderment."[35] That term comes from the adoptee rights movement, which has argued that losing access to one's heritage is damaging and unjust. If you don't have a friend or relative to donate sperm, you might seek out an intermediary, consultant, or company willing to recruit donors, as is common with egg donors and surrogates. You might run your own ad, targeted to your needs (for example, searching in your ethnic community), ask someone to do initial screening for your concerns, then refer potential donors to a sperm bank to be screened for you. In 1990 the Men's Resource Center in Amherst, Massachusetts, set up the Alternative Families Project to offer support and information to men helping single women and lesbian couples have access to DI.[36] Today fresh sperm is less in use, but the model of altruistically motivated donors willing to meet the requests of parents-to-be has strong appeal. One drawback to recruiting a potential donor is that he may not pass medical screening, and if he does, frozen specimens will be quarantined, so delays or even dead-ends may lie ahead. But if you can't make your peace with sperm bank options and have ruled out asking someone you know, these approaches to donor recruitment may be worth the extra cost and time.

If You're Asking a Relative or Friend to Help

Parents-to-be asking someone they know for help have to deal with different unknowns, including the unknown reactions of everyone involved. At first you'll be uncertain whether or not he's willing, or able, to donate, a more complicated decision if he's married or in a committed relationship. Then you'll face decisions about how inseminations should be done, at home or with a doctor, with the recommended frozen sperm or fresh. As all of you learn about these options, you'll also be adjusting to a new role in your relationship with one another. Whereas anonymous donors have already been screened and their vials are ready for shipment, your relative or friend may be months away from helping you get started. Nevertheless, impatience or expedience can't rule your choices.

You may need some counseling. Couples often find the known donor decision and logistics very challenging. Reviewing your list of potential friends and relatives can quickly overwhelm you both. Some choices that seem logical to one of you might horrify the other. Men will sometimes consider their fathers, while a father-in-law would almost never be a wife's choice. Although insemination is as asexual an activity as imaginable, the incest taboo seems to get stirred up, especially with much younger relatives. A wife might argue for an anonymous donor, worrying about complications with her brother-in-law, while her husband feels he can only do DI with his family genes. It can take time to reach a mutually acceptable decision.

It's vital that you know your options before you ask someone to donate. You'll be teaching him about DI and assessing whether it seems like something he should proceed with. He needs to know you have other options, however unready you are to consider them. You can't pressure him, even if you're desperate and can't see any other alternatives.

By asking a friend or relative, you're setting yourself up for the possibility of rejection. You may see your request as giving your donor the ultimate compliment and the chance to give you the gift of a lifetime, but he might be frightened by the prospect of fathering a child who will not be "his." He needs time to think it through and space to say no if this isn't for him. One couple came to see Carol because the husband's brother kept putting them off, not saying no *exactly*, and the wife felt her husband couldn't admit how highly ambivalent his brother was. The brother had delayed them many months, afraid to refuse. You have to realistically assess how your request is affecting the other person.

Collaborative reproduction that involves a brother or friend is discussed much less than when it involves women donating eggs or carrying a pregnancy, so it's hard to learn how others have coped. In *Having Your Baby by Donor Insemination*, author Elizabeth Noble tells of the beliefs she shared with her husband, rejecting DI secrecy. She felt she couldn't carry a child without knowing the donor. In her book she presents arguments for known donors and against anonymous DI. But her subsequent divorce and later marriage to her donor, who updated their story in a 1995 article,[37] made many long for a model family far less complicated.

Tom Riordan's reactions to Noble's book while he and his wife were considering DI raises common concerns about known donors.

> Take Elizabeth Noble, for example. . . . When I began her book, I was immediately unsettled by the dedication on the first page: to her child and the donor, a friend of her husband's. "But where is her husband?" I worried. As I read through the book, I continued to worry. The husband seemed a minor figure. The inseminations she described with their known donor seemed very cloak-and-dagger, very romantic. The donor slipped into the bathroom during a party, produced his sperm, and then slipped out, unnoticed. Then Noble slipped in and inseminated herself. Again I wondered, "Where is her husband?" . . .
>
> In our case, it helped that Joanna is both introspective and honest. She told me that she wasn't sure, if we used a friend as a donor, that she wouldn't feel a connection with him that would cause ripples in our marriage. She said that she would want to feel some kind of intimate connection; that part of the advantage of having a known donor for her, was that she would be taking into her body the sperm of someone she knew and cared about, and not an anonymous stranger. And I was introspective and honest enough to say, "No, I wouldn't like that."
>
> Other reasons against using a known donor occurred to us later. . . . If Joanna didn't get pregnant, would that cast doubt back on the donor's fertility? If we asked someone to be a donor and he said no, would that wrinkle our relationship? How would the donor's wife handle the "intimate connection" that her husband now had with my wife? Or if they had no children of their own, how would they handle that? Enough to say, "No, I wouldn't like that."[38]

Creating scenarios, focusing on different events in the child's life and how each family member might then feel about the role of the "biological father," can help you envision whether these complexities are ones you're confident you can handle or ones you'd rather avoid.

Men often favor brothers as donors, but their reasons and approaches can vary. Most would agree that one advantage is carrying on their family line, if not their exact set of genes. Some feel that having their brother as donor is the best way to conceal DI, and ask him to keep donating a secret, sometimes from everyone else in the family. Others feel it will make telling their child easier because there won't be any unknowns and, in fact, most biological relationships will remain the same; for example, the paternal grandparents would be grandparents genetically. As Susan McDaniel, a family therapist, expresses it, "Projecting into the future, these solutions allow the child to know his or her biological parent and know that the gift was given in love rather than casually or for money."[39] Laney writes:

> Both brothers wanted to help us, so we said we'd accept this very special gift from them. Somehow it would be a family effort. If and when we were successful in producing a child, the paternity would be known and shared with the family. It felt awkward and a little embarrassing at times to be having a planning session with my husband's brothers about how I was to have a baby. At least his parents weren't included at this point! There's cohesiveness, a lot of love and generosity and acceptance in his family. We all felt a comfort and sense that it would work, that we could deal with whatever came up, now or in the future.

Neither the known nor anonymous donor approach is simple or problem-free. Just as couples must learn to check in with each other about DI feelings over the years of parenting, so they must learn to talk with the brother about his feelings over time, and with his partner. By involving family members, some anxieties surrounding anonymous DI, such as the child's appearance, the donor's background, or the child's search for his roots someday, become moot. As Marie explains, "Because it was Ed's brother, I was able to dispel a lot of the mystery surrounding an unknown donor, which I think helped us concentrate on other things."

On the other hand, anonymous donors may be easier or wiser for some people. Karen agreed to using Joseph's four brothers' sperm with trepidation. After those inseminations didn't work, they went on to anonymous DI. She remembers:

> At first with my brothers-in-law, it felt kind of weird. After every insemination I'd try to imagine which brother it was and what the baby would look like, since I knew what they looked like. When I used the donor, I never really thought about what the child would look like.

The most difficult step may be the very first, raising the topic with your brother or friend. Perhaps he has known of your longing for a child and has offered—or whose name has been put forth by someone else in your family or circle of friends. But usually you'll be asking someone whose first reaction may be disbelief, maybe like yours when you first heard about DI. He and his partner need to understand not only the immediate requirements medically but also your hopes and expectations for the years of family life ahead. Anne and Larry recall that selecting a donor was much like selecting a husband, but "with none of the romance." In asking her friend, Anne remembers explaining to him:

> Larry and I wanted to have a baby, but Larry had had a vasectomy. So we were looking for a donor. And would he consider it? I remember trying to tell him that we'd want the baby to know him and . . . for him to be involved with her. I remember hoping I wasn't scaring him off.

Anne's friend accepted and continues to be part of their family, called "Papa John" by their daughter. Anne offers this advice:

> When you've asked your potential donor, it's time to spin out some scenarios again, this time in your trio. How much will you tell, and to whom,

and when? How much a part of the family will the donor be? Are there things about which strong conflict can be anticipated (like religious conflicts or parenting styles or educational expectations)? Not that you can really predict, but it's helpful to try to imagine points of decision so you can see if you are all three imagining the same kind of relationship.

Not all of this has to happen the first time you talk. Sandy writes that her donor was not only willing to participate but "seemed flattered to be involved and he wanted to be the guardian to the child." That may be a good point at which to take a break and let your donor go off and think things over.

You must be clear about how open or private you're planning to be. Erin, living in France and commuting to New York for inseminations after she and her husband asked his brother to be their donor, has been very open. "Society doesn't condone known donors . . . the comments we've gotten! I must admit I get a lot of pleasure from seeing people's reactions and then the ensuing discussion." But not everyone thrives on the controversy, and your donor-to-be might even be shaken by it. If he feels the need to have a confidant who can help him reach a solid decision more effectively, you may want to have some input into who that person is. You want someone who is objective, not biased against DI with a known donor. If you wish to keep your inner circle small, you can tell him who already knows and ask him to talk to only these confidants. You can also seek out an infertility counselor to help him consider your request.

Once you talk as a family or with your friend, you also need to find a medical team comfortable with DI with a known donor. Marie recalls:

> I brought up the idea of DI with a known donor (Ed's brother), and to my surprise the doctor quickly tried to dismiss the whole idea. "Oh, you don't want to do that. What if there's a family fight someday, when everyone is together? . . . No, no . . . you don't want to do that, then you'll need a lawyer to make sure you're never sued for custody. . . ." He

was very "anti" this. I told him my husband's family is different, they wouldn't do that, they're more into helping than hurting each other . . . but again, this doctor sort of brushed the idea away and said he wouldn't perform that type of procedure. We'd have to see someone else.

They did go ahead and ask his brother, who accepted without hesitation, saying, "Sure, I'd be honored." They did follow that doctor's advice to draw up a legal agreement, to clarify for professionals that there would be no lawsuits or custody battles.

Legal advice is important with known donors. For married couples it might only clarify agreements, such as his promise to provide medical updates. There are legal risks for unmarried women, however, that need to be addressed. If your child is someday in need, your donor might be found responsible for meeting those needs if you can't. If your donor ever wants more involvement than you agreed to, the absence of a dad might give him power. You want clear intent that he is a known donor, not a dad.

The next step is to begin discussing the realities of fertility treatment and insemination with your donor-to-be. He'll have questions about what's expected of him, and for some of them you may only be able to say, "I'm not sure yet, but I'll find out." If you've already located your doctor, you may want to arrange for your donor to meet the medical team. He will also need to meet with the sperm bank staff if you plan to have his sperm frozen.

One of the toughest realities is that his life, especially his sex life, will be under scrutiny as he becomes a donor. To maximize sperm counts, he shouldn't ejaculate for a day or two before each donation. Even during your decision-making stage, you'll need to know that he's been practicing "safe sex." This is especially true if your donor is gay or bisexual, even though he may have been more careful than heterosexuals. Anne writes about considering John. "I needed to say to him, 'My life is in your hands' and hear him say that he knew that and wouldn't do anything to endanger either of our lives or the life of our baby." A brother or friend might learn, because of your screening, that he, too, is infertile.

While your known donor heads off to think, or to be screened, you can be learning more about what you'll need to get started with inseminations.

GETTING STARTED WITH YOUR CHOSEN DONOR

Getting started may now be a very rapid process for you, presenting few challenges beyond those you've already faced. If you quickly become pregnant, your initial donor choice may be your only one lifelong.

However, this isn't always the way DI goes. It may be difficult to learn, after all your work on donor selection, that you may change your choice in the weeks or months ahead. The reason for the change may be under your control: you decide that some characteristic or quality is more important to you than you'd realized, for example, or you discover new resources such as a sperm bank you hadn't heard of earlier. But you may change for more frustrating reasons: your first-choice donor has no specimens available, or your brother begins to feel uncomfortable with donating. But if you get off to a good start, future choices will be easier.

•

We've covered a lot of ground in this chapter. You might think that you don't have to invest so much energy in choosing a donor, that you'll love your child no matter which vial you choose. That's certainly true. But remember, with any luck your donor will be the biological parent of your child. We don't get to pick our parents . . . but here you do get to pick some of your child's genes. It's worth a little extra effort.

Chapter Four

Getting Started

It was a forty-five-minute drive to the NYC doctor we then were sure was the best around. Amazingly, I got a parking place right out front, so it must have been a weekend. I remember the doctor coming into the exam room and telling us how he'd prepared the specimen for freezing with his own new egg yolk protectant, better than what anybody else was using. We were both nervous, not quite knowing what to expect. Overall, it was anticlimactic. I remember the speculum, and the cervical cap that was a bit painful for Heidi. I was there to hold Heidi's hand the whole time she was stuck on her back with her legs in the air. We can't remember if I said, "Go, spermies, go," as I had early on whenever we made love, before my diagnosis; I think I did. We went out to a great ice cream place afterward. We spent the day together, and when we went home, we curled up together while we talked about it. After that first time, the medical process didn't seem like a big deal to me, although I know that emotionally it was always more than routine for Heidi.

—*Bob*

Getting started with donor insemination presents a new set of choices. Even the simplest decisions—who should order the sperm or how to schedule an insemination—may be unclear. You may be worried about how much time, effort, and cost you'll be facing once you finally get started. You'll need some help to understand

93

your options and to decide on the approach that will get you off to a good start, medically and emotionally. Sometimes there won't be many choices—for example, if only one doctor in your area offers DI. Some decisions you may defer to your medical team. But you do need to clarify your wishes, for yourself, for your health care providers, and for those you will turn to for support.

You may become pregnant the first month, although statistics say that *most* couples do not. You can have a successful cycle emotionally, if not medically, if you can learn about your reactions, reconfirm your decision, and clarify what support you need. You may find the first cycle very difficult and realize that you need to spend some time figuring out which of your early decisions didn't turn out as you'd expected or hoped. One couple learned they needed more time before beginning.

> The night before we were to go, we got cold feet. . . . What kind of person would donate sperm? How close a match would they do? . . . We were frightened when really faced with it. We were up all night trying to sort out our feelings. Finally I asked my husband if he would like more time, and he said yes. So we postponed for a month and hashed out many of our problems and concerns with the doctor, who was most supportive and understanding.[1]

Once you're ready, you'll learn a lot as you go through that first cycle.

Putting Together Your Medical Team

Who will help you make all the decisions about how to begin inseminations? Try to image a team approach. Most people would think of the doctor as the team leader, but it may be wiser to think of appointing a team leader as each task arises. That leader can focus on the task at hand with awareness of your needs. Sometimes only you can be in charge of the task, for example, asking someone you know to donate. Sometimes your infertility counselor will take on a central role, coaching you through a decision-making process as a couple. At some stages a sperm bank professional may play a large part, helping you narrow down donor choices. And, of course, your doctor will take on major responsibilities, with your input, in deciding how to increase your chances of becoming pregnant. The doctor's nursing staff may do many of your procedures, and their emotional sensitivity as well as technical expertise can make a big difference in your DI experience. Even the medical billing person who maximizes your coverage plays a vital role. Ultimately, parents-to-be should be the team managers, with veto power and final say.

DI often requires choosing new professionals for your team, which can be frustrating if you've already seen more doctors than you could ever have imagined. Some couples already in fertility treatment decide to stay put, satisfied with their care or reluctant to take any more time switching doctors. Others may need to find a specialist who does DI, generally a gynecologist with a strong interest in infertility or fellowship training in reproductive endocrinology. RESOLVE or the American Society for Reproductive Medicine can suggest specialists, or you can ask a local gynecologist to help you get started with DI, even if you later need to switch to someone more specialized.

If you have a number of physicians to choose from, what should you look for in a medical practice?

- Find an *infertility specialist* recommended by patients and consumer organizations such as RESOLVE or Single Mothers by Choice. Ask about their approach to donor insemination. You can also ask about their DI success rates if they keep them, but collecting this data isn't required, as it is for in vitro fertilization (IVF) and other assisted reproductive technologies (ARTs).

- Make sure *the staff is attuned to your specific requests or concerns.* Outline these in writing before your first consultation or as you become aware of an issue. Having your concerns in writing will increase the likelihood that any agreements about how to meet your needs will be placed in your chart and noticed by the staff at future visits.

- Work with a medical practice allowing a *diversity of donor options*. Some practices order from only one bank or promote their own affiliated bank. This could leave you wondering if there might have been a better donor match elsewhere.

- Make sure you're comfortable with their *approach to timing ovulation*. Testing can be simple or sophisticated, as we'll discuss later. If you're ovulating naturally, you may want to avoid any fertility drugs. DI patients used to be given clomiphene because it might "regulate" ovulation so that inseminations could be more easily scheduled. Nowadays clomiphene is seldom used unless ovulatory irregularity has been documented.

- Staff must be *skilled in intrauterine insemination* (IUI). As discussed later in this chapter, IUI is often preferable to intracervical insemination (ICI), but it requires some added expertise. Some practices do start with intracervical insemination, but if you turn out to need IUI, switching doctors after a couple of ICI cycles will be frustrating.

- *Weekend coverage* is important. If you ovulate on Saturday, you can't wait for a Monday insemination. Seven-day coverage is standard for ART programs. Even small practices sometimes have a sympathetic nurse or doctor willing to come in briefly for weekend inseminations.

- Access to *affordable sperm storage* facilities, on-site or nearby, can save you lots. Frozen sperm is shipped in liquid nitrogen tanks, which aren't cheap for the bank to get to your doctor—this is not a small UPS package! If there's a local sperm bank, you can save on shipping charges by picking up your specimens in one of these transport tanks. If your doctor has an on-site storage tank (doctors working with frozen embryos always do), you can save by shipping several vials at once. If you become pregnant, extra vials can then be stored for the future.

- A *good billing person* can get as much insurance reimbursement as procedure codes allow.

- A *primary contact* can help you identify any problems or needs.

Many couples are amazed that the medical team can be so matter-of-fact about such profound beginnings. For you DI is not routine, and doctor consultations may stir up memories of prior bad news, if not full-fledged trauma. Pam reports on her reaction after her first consult:

> Even though the doctor was nice enough, I get so damned depressed whenever I'm in those cold, sterile hospital rooms with nothing on but a piece of linen and my feet in stirrups. Not just that, it's hearing all the things they have to say in order to cover themselves in case of failure, like referring to my age and encouraging me to have an HSG [hysterosalpingo-gram, a dye X-ray of the uterine cavity and fallopian tubes] before I try even one insemination. I told the doctor I wanted to try the first cycle, three cycles actually, with just intrauterine insemination before considering the test. I would just feel more comfortable, more hopeful, doing it this way. She will suggest to my nurse-practitioner [at the referring HMO] that we do the HSG first, and I will talk with my nurse-practitioner about it.
>
> All the talk about these tests and possibly drugs in the future really got me down, brought all my grief back. Here is the first time that I finally get to try to become pregnant and then to go back to that sterile environment again with all the same old negative statistics. I thought that I was a strong, healthy woman! With the blood tests that they need to have done on me, and then meeting with my nurse-practitioner again, and then meeting with another nurse-practitioner who handles talking to us specifically about DI and the inseminations. . . . It looks like it will be longer than I had hoped before we can try.

REQUIRED COUNSELING

At some point you may be asked to meet with a psychotherapist before getting started. Although many feel this required visit is just another hoop to jump through, it does offer you a confidential place with a knowledgeable adviser to explore how you're coping with the DI decision. The goal is also to protect your doctor against claims that you were unprepared. Doctors must inform patients of possible negative outcomes of DI, and since some risks are psychological and marital, this gets delegated to counselors.

Take advantage and use the counseling sessions for your own goals. Organize a list of your remaining concerns. You can ask to return to a counselor who already knows you or to see someone with DI expertise. There are sometimes advantages to meeting with an on-site or affiliated counselor, who can intervene with your medical team with special requests or in a crisis.

While some people beginning DI rely on their inner circle for a deeper level of support, it can help to have a counselor on call. You'll be creating your safety net for the stressful weeks or months ahead.

PRELIMINARY MEDICAL TESTING

Before getting started, your doctor will review your records and perhaps run tests to see if any "female factors" are likely to affect DI treatment. For couples this raises the specter that even your second choice might not work, that both of you may be infertile. But early tests can detect minor, easily treated fertility problems. Medical recommendations on what tests to do before starting vary. What might be recommended for a twenty-five-year-old with no gynecological symptoms is different from what would be appropriate for a forty-year-old with endometriosis symptoms. Most doctors take into account your strong preferences, whether you want testing to let you know everything seems OK or whether you want to avoid testing that seems unnecessary.

One of the frequently upsetting tests is the one for HIV, which is done on both the husband and the wife. Its main purpose is to protect the doctor and the sperm bank, which could be accused of giving someone AIDS when in fact the person had already contracted HIV before DI.

AWAITING OVULATION

Since the lifetime of the egg after ovulation is quite short, it's important to pinpoint the time of ovulation accurately. If you haven't been in fertility treatment before, it can be very anxiety-provoking to wonder how to tell if you're ovulating. The most common method is an ovulation detection kit. Urine testing kits have replaced the daily ritual of basal body temperature (BBT) charting. Some women have insurance coverage for blood tests for LH (luteinizing hormone), ultrasounds to look for a follicle ready to release an egg, or a pelvic exam to check the cervical mucus. Few policies cover the cost of donor sperm itself, so tests to be sure you aren't "wasting" specimens on the wrong day are cost-effective. Some women feel reassured to have confirmation from the very start that everything looks normal.

TWO METHODS OF INSEMINATION

Inseminations can be intracervical (ICI) or intrauterine (IUI). ICI specimens go just inside the cervical opening, leaving the sperm to make their way through the cervical mucus, into the uterus, and out to the tubes. IUI inseminations are done with a thin, flexible catheter, which is passed through the cervix and into the uterus before the sperm are gently released. ICI is less expensive, both for the specimen and for the procedure. ICI is so simple that you can do home inseminations if you wish. Also, ICI is less likely to push other organisms into the uterus, where infection could do damage.

IUI seems to have a much higher success rate.[2] IUI helps specimens with lower motility (where the sperm might not be strong enough to travel the distance from the cervix to the egg) by placing the sperm beyond the cervical mucus. If the mucus isn't ideal, IUI also helps. If you've already ovulated, IUI can help the sperm get to the egg within the brief window of time when it can be fertilized, twelve to twenty-four hours after ovulation.[3] Since you won't know about these factors beforehand, you may want to plan on IUI so that your medical team isn't juggling at the last minute.

Before sperm can be placed in the uterus, they must be prepared, or "washed." Sperm cells with good motility, the ability to swim forward at a decent speed, are separated from other substances in the semen, such as prostaglandins, which can cause severe cramping.

Sometimes you choose ICI or IUI for a cycle because your chosen donor's sperm is available in only one type of vial that month. Let's say you want to get started and use your first-choice donor, but only ICI vials are available. If your doctor's office isn't equipped or staffed to get an ICI specimen prepped for IUI, which happens on weekends particularly, you'll probably need to accept ICI for this cycle.

If you order IUI-ready specimens, already processed at the sperm bank before freezing, you'll pay more for the specimen but not need processing at your doctor's office. One study found this more cost-effective.

> Typically, to obtain the number of motile sperm provided in the IUI-ready specimen, it is necessary to process two vials of frozen semen. The cost of the second vial, plus the cost of local processing, increases patient cost to more than double the cost of the IUI-ready specimen with current pricing structures. Hence, we conclude that use of IUI-ready donor semen specimens from a commercial laboratory, at the present time, offers significant economic benefit to the patient without compromising the IUI pregnancy rate.[4]

Ordering three or four vials can save you months of effort, although the initial cost will be high. Ben writes about their very first (and successful!) cycle:

> Our lab technician said we'd only need two; Dr. S. said we'd better order three. We ordered four. That was about three weeks ago. My wife got a positive OvuQuick result on a Thursday and went in for IUI the next day, but the ultrasound showed no ovulation yet. Then, on Saturday, the

same thing happened. The doctor gave my wife an hCG shot. Sunday, again no ovulation. We had natural home insemination. Monday, finally, ultrasound revealed she had ovulated. The IUI was done, but the lab found one of the donor vials was a poor sample. So all four got used. Good thing we had them available.

The cost of ordering "extra" sperm paid off in the reward of rapid success. If you don't use every vial, storing extras locally may be cheaper than monthly shipping charges.

Trying to "hit" the time of ovulation, many physicians suggest two inseminations, spaced a day apart, whereas others do just one well-timed insemination. You should have some say in this. For example, your job may not welcome absences so close together. But sometimes a second insemination is necessary, especially if you hadn't yet ovulated before the first. Sometimes if the mucus isn't good on the day of an ICI, you can come back for IUI-prepped sperm, which can bypass that mucus.

TESTS EVEN WHILE YOU WAIT FOR NEWS

Waiting to see if you're pregnant may be a welcome break. But your doctor might recommend you use even this first cycle to check on your fertility and correct any minor problems in the second half of the cycle, the luteal phase. About a week after insemination, a blood test can predict if your level of progesterone is high enough to keep the uterine lining ready for a fertilized egg to implant. If the progesterone level is low, natural progesterone can be given orally, as a vaginal suppository, or by injection.

Some practices will also draw blood for pregnancy testing, especially if your period is at all late. An early positive test proves that sperm got to the egg. Many early pregnancies do miscarry, at least 25 percent of all pregnancies. This doesn't necessarily mean there's any additional fertility problem. Initial positive news is often called a "chemical pregnancy" until about three weeks later, when a heartbeat can be seen on ultrasound. While it's sad to know you lost a beginning pregnancy, the information can lead to preventive steps, such as extra progesterone, in your next cycle.

But You Wanted a Low-Key Beginning?

You may have hoped to begin DI in a low-key way that wouldn't get you anxious about everything that could go wrong. If everything looks fine (you ovulate, have good mucus, and so on), starting off with minimal medical intervention is an option. You may want to predict ovulation simply (and more cheaply), skipping ultrasound and blood work for a home ovulation-predictor kit. You may ask for only one insemination, especially if you travel a distance or have job difficulties. You may wish to start with whatever insemination procedure your medical practice feels is simplest, and hope for the best this first time.

Some people want to "demedicalize" the process with home inseminations. Home insemination has been most common when asking a brother or friend to donate and using fresh sperm, because often doctors are unwilling to assist with fresh sperm. The Sperm Bank of California began teaching home insemination because many single women and lesbian couples couldn't find specialists willing to treat them. Some practices teach home insemination techniques for weekends. Some couples just find insemination easier to deal with at home. Alison writes about trying home insemination after her husband's failed vasectomy reversal led to DI.

> The first time was very emotionally charged. I cried by myself the night before in the bathroom at the thought of what we were doing. . . . We wanted to do the inseminations ourselves, so I found a nurse-midwife who received the sperm for us and we did the inseminations at home. I really recommend that approach for people without female infertility problems. It was so intimate and so an act of love—so different from the IUIs months later.

WHEN YOU'D RATHER NOT START SLOWLY

Sometimes starting slowly feels like a waste of time. Some women know they need medication to help ovulation. For others the decision is uncertain—cycles are long or kits never quite turn color or temperature charts never look perfect. You may want to learn about options to enhance ovulation right from the start.

You also have the option to monitor specimen quality. Most banks have policies on minimum standards. But a refund doesn't undo a missed cycle. You may need to switch donors if specimens don't thaw out well, so you need warning of that problem.

YOUR EMOTIONAL NEEDS AT THAT FIRST INSEMINATION

While you're working with your medical team toward optimal chances for a pregnancy, you'll want optimal emotional conditions too. Unfortunately, insemination procedures may be easier to figure out than what each of you needs emotionally. Neither spouse can guess how the other is going to react to these never-imagined steps toward pregnancy. Many women don't look forward to sharing their time in the stirrups with anyone but the required medical staff. But this visit may lead to your baby's conception, and many couples want to be together for such a crucial event. The first insemination can be confusing or sad. Anne writes:

> My first IUI, using Clomid, was the most difficult. Though Clyde was with me, holding my hand, I felt as if I was being unfaithful to him by using another man's sperm, in spite of the fact that our pregnancy efforts were quite clinical.

Humor can help, as Leigh recalls.

> I didn't think about what was going on until I had to lie down (tilted) for 20 minutes. I was nervous . . . then I thought of the movie *Look Who's*

> *Talking*—in the beginning, it shows sperm swimming up the fallopian tubes to the Beach Boys' song "I Get Around" and Bruce Willis's voice is saying, "This way, guys, around the corner . . ." It helped break the tension.

For some, insemination is an anticlimax. Becki reports:

> At first I was afraid it would feel weird (emotionally, not physically) to be inseminated with another man's sperm. But we had already been going through inseminations with Steve's sperm for about a year, and the procedure was the same. And Steve was the one there with me, holding my hand. Emotionally, we both just felt excited that we might be creating a life.

Some couples wonder whether to make love around the time of insemination. For some this is a powerful symbol of connection. For others, lovemaking on schedule is only stressful, so a dinner out or a walk holding hands might better express your commitment. Sherry writes:

> I was inseminated two or three times per month. After each insemination, our doctor advised us to go home and make love. He called it "doing your homework." The purpose of this, he said, was so we would never really know if a pregnancy was the result of the donor sperm or if, by some miracle, one of my husband's sperm had hit the mark. This suggestion was offered, I suppose, as comfort, but the love we made after inseminations felt mechanical and inept, like running behind a bulldozer while brandishing a spoon. Often we felt vaguely absurd.[5]

Thomas and Ellen learned a medical reason to avoid intercourse after insemination, but only after six unsuccessful cycles. At their seventh all the donor sperm were found dead on the second day of inseminations. After learning of the very high level of sperm antibodies in his semen, Thomas joked, "Not only can I not make my wife pregnant, but I'm keeping anyone else from making her pregnant as well!" He made sure to wear a condom, another ironic chapter in their infertility saga.

STARTING WITH A KNOWN DONOR

Getting started with a brother or friend as your donor brings different challenges, particularly if his sperm hasn't been frozen and home insemination seems like the most feasible route. With their friend John donating sperm, Anne and Larry had to learn insemination techniques.

> I didn't have any feelings about "being inseminated" because it wasn't a passive process. I was the one doing the inseminating. The actual physical process of inserting the cervical cap was a bit intimidating at first—I probably should have practiced well in advance with some KY jelly or something in the cap. But it got easier over time. . . . Though Larry and I discussed the possibility of my going to visit John by myself, we always went together. I think it was better that way. It would have been strange to get pregnant with Larry in another state.

Others feel more confident proceeding if they can find a physician willing to be involved, rare given the professional guidelines for freezing and quarantining. Marie's physician helped coordinate inseminations with her brother-in-law. After thorough testing to be sure no one currently tested positive for any sexually transmittable infections, all three had to sign waivers stating that they understood the risks of transmitting undetected infections, particularly HIV, in fresh sperm.

The logistics of inseminating with fresh sperm can be horrendous as you try to link your schedule to your donor's. Erin found the commute from Paris to New York, where her brother-in-law was living, didn't help their stress level when getting started.

> I have so far tried two cycles and both have failed. . . . This has not been easy for us. . . . I am trying to figure out a way to stop flying over the ocean. . . . The twist on DI here in France is that it is illegal to use sperm from someone you know.

Even when you are the one doing the traveling, there's the added pressure of fearing you are inconveniencing your donor and that he'll back out. You may do everything you can, be accommodating to an absurd level, to get his sperm to your doctor with as little hassle as possible for him. Marie rushed from her brother-in-law's job site with that special delivery—and got stopped by a state cop for speeding! Not only does your life revolve around ovulation, but you must also worry if your donor can learn to live this way.

With incredible distances or scheduling complexities, your brother or friend can work with a sperm bank. He'll be screened as a "directed" donor, his specimens permanently held just for your use. At one visit one specimen can be divided into several vials if his sperm quality is good. Once out of quarantine, vials can be shipped to your specialist. The start-up costs and delays can save in the long run, especially if you're planning more than one pregnancy.

Reacting to Your First Cycle

People often revert to old habits under stress. If one of you retreats with the TV remote control and the other wants to talk over every detail, it's not easy. It's wise to cut out as many other stresses as possible and add in more of whatever helps you feel supported in tough times.

While so much of the focus falls on husbands during the decision-making stage, this stage can put a great deal of pressure on women. Chris remembers, "I now felt anxious that the infertility spotlight was off John and on me, with the expectation that good results would be forthcoming." Everyone has to deal with the suspense of waiting. Leigh felt it from the day of her first insemination. "Another long two-week wait ahead. I'll try to keep busy so I don't think about it twenty-four hours a day—but that is pretty much impossible!"

While you wait for the results of your first cycle, you can evaluate how the process went for you. You may decide to both take the day off for any future inseminations. You may want to set up a consultation with your doctor to clear up confusion. You may decide to pick another donor if the current profile didn't feel quite right. You may need to wait on a second cycle until you can cut down on stress in other areas of your life.

Occasionally a couple goes through a crisis during the first cycle, even when they both thought they were ready. Cindy was interviewed years later for an article on living without children.

> At 37, Cindy thought, maybe she should rethink her aversion to donor insemination. . . . They tried one cycle of donor insemination, in Jim's words, "a very bold thing for us because we're very conservative." Then, Cindy says, "I suddenly started to really panic that I could be pregnant with someone else's child. I was almost devastated." "I had feelings that it's not going to be mine, and I'm going to be outside the whole thing," Jim says. "When Cindy panicked it was a relief." It was a relief, too, when she was not pregnant.[6]

Jim and Cindy were fortunate that they realized simultaneously that DI wasn't the best alternative for them. For many couples the reaction of one will be very threatening or angering to the other. It can feel like an overwhelming step backward to look again at your decision and reconsider other alternatives. Some feel a great deal of pain during their first cycle but see it as a reaction they're able to work through before trying again.

One crisis that can be both joyful and frightening is triggered when the very first cycle leads to a pregnancy. You thought this was a trial run, and now you're facing the real thing. Eric was in shock when Lisa's period was late.

> I kept on saying that it couldn't be. Dr. W. had said it hardly ever works the first time. In my heart, I was hoping that there still was a chance for me. This donor was just a fly-by-night. . . . I couldn't believe that after I couldn't do it in over two years, this guy could do it in two "beef jerky" injections![7]

Eric's feelings were more positive when testing confirmed the news. "The whole world stopped. I just sat there and froze and then cried. I was so happy, I didn't stop grinning for a week!"[8]

For better or worse, most don't get pregnant so quickly. If you're just starting, we hope you'll soon be skipping ahead to the pregnancy chapter. But if DI is becoming frustrating, the next chapter may help you feel less alone during the Trying Times.

Chapter Five

Trying Times: When Donor Insemination Takes Its Time

After five months of DI, Bob was tired of waiting and ready to start toward adoption too. At that point we still hadn't spoken to anyone who'd gotten pregnant using DI. And it obviously wasn't going to work for us, as far as Bob was concerned. He's the type who likes instant gratification and expected DI to work quickly. I wasn't ready to give up, which left me feeling that I'd better get pregnant fast or I'd end up doing something I wasn't ready for.

It was month seven and our patience was wearing thin and our tempers were short. On day 11 I was getting pains like I do when I ovulate, but over the past six months my ovulation kit had faithfully turned blue between day 14 and 18. When I told Bob I wanted to start ovulation testing, he was frustrated because "wasting" three days would mean we'd need to buy two kits. I still did the test, and it turned blue. I remember jumping around the apartment, teasing him, saying, "I was right and you were wrong!" And wrong he was; our son was born nine months later. I still get goose bumps realizing we wouldn't have our son if I'd missed that ovulation. The frustration of trying and the fear of stressing Bob any further almost kept me from listening to my body and trusting my intuition.

—Heidi

One myth about donor insemination is that it quickly leads to pregnancy. When that doesn't happen, anxiety can build quickly. Emotional, medical, and financial difficulties that you had assumed would be short-lived can seem overwhelming. There are many steps you can take to optimize your chances for pregnancy, but these can take you from a low-key beginning to the most high-tech methods reproductive medicine has to offer. Achieving a pregnancy via DI requires that you and your medical team beat the odds stacked against you each cycle as you try to get frozen sperm, with its less-than-perfect motility, to a mature egg via a medical procedure that has to be performed within the brief window of time during which a mature egg can be fertilized each month.

You may begin to realize that you do need to learn more about the fertility treatment options that can increase your chances of DI working, many of which we'll outline later in this chapter. You may also begin to seriously consider the other two major alternatives to continuing with medical treatment. One alternative is adding to your family via adoption. Another is to end your attempts to add to your family by resolving to live without children or, for those facing DI after secondary infertility, to live as a one-child family.

It takes courage and determination to continue making these decisions. Sometimes the ongoing grind of the Trying Times becomes terribly depressing, frustrating, or infuriating. And sometimes there are events that are more than trying—they are tragic—as you receive the terrible news of a miscarriage, of untreatable female infertility factors, of the end of your dream of a pregnancy via this alternative you worked so hard to begin.

Some of the stories in this chapter have the happy ending of a pregnancy. Some have a different resolution through adoption or child-free living. Some are sagas that continue with no clear end in sight. We'll help you anticipate how you could cope with difficult medical decisions, consider when enough is enough, and move on to other alternatives. As you prepare to cope with the worst, you don't need to give up hope for much better. Your next cycle may bring the happy news that you're leaving the Trying Times behind.

WORKING TOWARD PREGNANCY

There are many reasons DI doesn't work quickly. Maybe your number hasn't come up yet, because even at the peak of fertility, pregnancy rates are only about 25 percent per cycle. Age-related drops in fertility rates have been reported in scientific journals[1] and by the media. The odds of getting pregnant even in a well-timed intrauterine insemination (IUI) cycle are probably about the same as rolling a six—only there is a lot more riding on this roll!

You have more control over other factors that can lower your chances further. Highly motile sperm must reach an egg within a small window of time after ovulation. DI at the wrong time offers a 0 percent chance. In this chapter we'll help you learn to work with your medical team to coordinate your ovulation with their insemination procedures. You need to understand what options exist to optimize DI treatment.

You may have to consider the possibility of female fertility problems too. The odds of any couple's both having reduced fertility aren't really as rare as lightning striking twice. Couples who have faced severe male infertility factors must remember that the wife's "subfertility" or "impaired fertility" may be very treatable. Even the most minor problem can be significant when frozen sperm is used. Women may have to accept that they'll need some tests and treatment too. If you have a more serious problem, such as tubal damage, you may face tough choices, such as surgical repair or turning to in vitro fertilization (IVF) with donor sperm.

You need to become an active partner in managing your medical care. If you want to trust your medical team and be a "good patient," you should realize this isn't incompatible with active participation. You need to report any symptoms or history that might be clues to female fertility factors. Your help analyzing the last unsuccessful cycle can improve the odds for the next. You need to signal your team that you can be a player, that you don't need to sit on the sidelines, protected from the facts or spared stressful questions. Maybe you fear you'll be seen as second-guessing, interfering, or overreacting, but that's preferable to looking back on months of cooperative, polite trying that had little or no chance of working because some factor was overlooked.

You may fear you don't have enough understanding of fertility treatment even to ask good questions. And no one likes to feel stupid or helpless in front of sometimes intimidating medical professionals. But there is a good saying to remember—the only stupid question is the one you didn't ask. One logical approach to understanding your medical options is to move chronologically through the cycle, learning what might go wrong or could be better.

CHECKING FOR OPTIMAL OVULATION

If your ovulation hasn't been predictable or sometimes doesn't happen at all, your doctor will probably recommend some intervention in the first half of the cycle to be sure you have a mature egg waiting for insemination. Ovulation induction is as much an art as a science. Not only can ovulation be slightly off in several ways, but it can be off for you in one cycle and be fine the next. Infertility specialists try not to overtreat because fixing one factor, such as egg maturation, can throw off another, such as your uterine lining. The 1990s brought fears of side effects with ovulation-inducing drugs, and until long-term studies can clarify any risks, many doctors and patients are reluctant to use medication unnecessarily.

Ovulatory problems aren't unusual, however, and even a subtle difference in one hormone level can be a clue that treatment is needed. Some medications speed up egg development, important if a woman doesn't ovulate until several days beyond the "typical" day 14. Sometimes women need help releasing the ripened egg from the ovarian follicle. Some women need supplementation of one hormone, such as progesterone, in the second half of their cycle, or suppression of another hormone, such as prolactin.

The most well-known ovulatory medication is clomiphene, sold as Clomid or Serophene. In pill form it's often thought of as an easy way to encourage egg development. Yet you and your doctor need to be sure clomiphene's possible negative side effects don't outweigh its value. It's an antiestrogen, tricking the pituitary into producing more FSH (follicle-stimulating hormone) and LH (luteinizing hormone), which signal the ovaries to mature eggs. But its antiestrogenic side effects can make the cervical mucus or uterine lining less than ideal. And emotionally it can make women tearful or irritable. June writes:

> We did two cycles with Clomid and IUI. It was summer and the hot flashes were very hot! I could handle that, but the other side effect was depression. I wasn't sure if it was magnified by too much time with the infertility dragon. But I was an unhappy, very depressed cookie.

Many husbands would agree that it's good to avoid those side effects. But there are many clomiphene babies.

Clomiphene alone doesn't always help with the release of the mature egg. Some women don't produce the surge of LH that triggers egg release. Some have a cystic ovarian surface that makes it difficult for the follicle to follow the hormone's command to rupture. One injection of human chorionic gonadotropin (hCG, with the common brand names Profasi and Pregnyl) will mimic the pituitary's LH surge and improve chances of the egg's release, which occurs about thirty-six hours later.

Clomiphene is only the first approach to inducing ovulation, and if it hasn't worked after a few cycles, your doctor may suggest more advanced treatment with purified forms of the pituitary hormones, given by injection. The dosage for each evening's injection during the first half of your cycle, when eggs are maturing, is determined by a blood test done that morning. Ultrasounds of your ovaries will also help determine how the medication is affecting the development of the follicles, the fluid-filled sacs in which each egg floats. It is hard to believe that the tiny amounts of medication you dilute and draw up in a syringe each night can be so powerful—or expensive! Pergonal was the first brand of injectable gonadotropins to be widely used; the medication sold under the brand name Humegon also contains both FSH and LH. Metrodin, another standard medication, contains just FSH and thus has slightly different effects on egg development. Fertinex is the brand name of a medication released in 1996 that offers the advantage of easier injections with smaller syringes.

The brand names vary, but the purposes are similar. One purpose of these medications is to treat ovulatory problems that are serious enough to make a pregnancy unlikely otherwise. Some women seldom ovulate, some ovulate before the egg is fully matured, and some develop multiple small cysts. With creative combinations of medications, doctors try to fine-tune ovulation. Another common purpose is to shorten the Trying Times by developing more than one egg, referred to as controlled ovarian hyperstimulation (COH). When using this method with reproductive technologies such as IVF, the medical team removes the eggs and freezes the extra embryos for future attempts. But insemination when several eggs have been ovulated can put you at risk for multiple embryos' implanting. So you need to discuss the pros and cons of this treatment with your doctor.

Treatment doesn't stop at ovulation. Progesterone is needed in the correct amount to make the uterine lining receptive to implanting by an embryo. There are tests that can detect progesterone abnormalities. And once you're using medications for egg development, it's assumed the uterine lining needs some help. Fortunately, natural progesterone is available in a number of forms.

Many other female fertility factors can interfere with DI. Endometriosis, uterine defects as minor as a polyp, or immunity problems are common examples. There are other illnesses, such as thyroid disease or diabetes, that have an impact on fertility. Don't hesitate to ask your medical team about your medical history or unusual symptoms. Ask other specialists you've seen for seemingly unrelated problems to research possible fertility effects. Most problems can be helped or bypassed, so don't be afraid to find out what female factors could be slowing things down.

Are Healthy Sperm Getting to That Mature Egg?

Any treatment with ovulation-inducing drugs is usually followed by intrauterine insemination (if not a more high-tech ART). The reasons for IUI were outlined in the last chapter. If you've chosen a "perfect" donor but the specimens don't look ideal after the lab's usual sperm wash, it's worth asking the lab to compare different IUI prep methods to see which works best with your donor's specimens.[2]

When to do your insemination is another controversy. Studies of insemination procedures have used different methods to detect ovulation and then different insemination timings in relation to that presumed ovulation time.[3] Some believe careful timing is vital because of the shortened life span of frozen sperm. Since sperm must be in the fallopian tubes around the time of the egg's arrival, and since the egg can only be fertilized for twelve to twenty-four hours, these experts conclude that you benefit from pinpointing ovulation as closely as possible.[4] But one study compared four different methods of detecting ovulation and found that all worked equally well if insemination was within twenty-four hours of the predicted ovulation[5].

Your medical team can work with you to pick a feasible way to pinpoint ovulation and to schedule your insemination(s) around that. If you're using a urine testing kit, you can test every twelve hours instead of daily when you're close to your usual day. Luteinizing hormone (LH), which triggers ovulation, is released in a sudden surge, so your morning test could be negative but by evening the surge might have begun. Ultrasound can show if a follicle has reached the size typical for mature eggs or has already burst. If you've had an egg-releasing shot of hCG because your kit never changed color or because you're using medications routinely combined with hCG, your doctor can make a good guess about your time of ovulation, usually thirty-six hours after the injection.

Once you understand what you need—ultrasound, IUI, and so on— you may need both persistence and charm to get everything optimally scheduled. It's wise to work with a nurse or medical secretary who knows the plan and can set up whatever you need. Barbara would bring coffee from Dunkin Donuts to her ultrasonographer as part of their "deal" to get ultrasounds done a half hour early so that she could get to work on time and avoid angering her boss. Sometimes staff aren't so accommodating, but if you can tell that they're stressed too, you may feel less resentful of their not making DI easier for you. Nevertheless, many couples feel overlooked while attention goes to high-tech procedures. Patty went in for a weekend insemination and was told no one was available for her IUI because they were busy with IVF patients.

The specimen's quality obviously affects your chances for pregnancy in a cycle. You can ask your medical team about each specimen. One study noted high per-cycle pregnancy rates (27 percent) if motility remained over 50 percent, despite the damaging effects of freezing.[6] Another study noted high pregnancy rates (31 percent) if there were more than 100 million sperm.[7] Less-than-ideal specimens are upsetting, but at least you'll have some explanation if a cycle doesn't lead to pregnancy.

Some physicians sidestep controversies about sufficient numbers by using two vials per insemination. You may say it's worth every penny if it speeds up your pathway to pregnancy and gets you out of the Trying Times. But until it does, it is frustrating to wonder whether the specimen quality is a major part of why you aren't yet pregnant. And what if it isn't the donor, what if the specimens are really fine? Is the delay in pregnancy a sign of a problem with you? You and your medical team do need solid data to sort out these questions.

It sometimes is the donor. It's now understood that not all normal-appearing sperm fertilize eggs. As Arthur, now a DI dad, puts it, "I have lots of sperm and when we did IVF, we learned that they all swim around avoiding eggs like the plague. I have so many sperm I could go qualify as a donor, but my sperm do nothing." Most tests of fertilization potential, developed to diagnose male infertility, are costly or complicated to run and have uncertain accuracy. Sperm banks generally don't want to add that cost to the screening of each donor. And no matter how a specimen is analyzed, an actual pregnancy is still the only proof that a man's sperm can fertilize eggs. Ask if your donor's sperm has led to conceptions, either via DI or in his personal life (although the latter doesn't speak to possible problems due to freezing). William Byrd, the director of a Texas sperm bank, found that specimens from four of the twenty-five donors he studied never produced a pregnancy.

> The problem is that you might have the best-looking donor around, he's got a great sperm count, they're really kicking, he freezes well—but it turns out he's shooting blanks. The sperm just does not get women pregnant.[8]

And even a donor with good sperm can have a bad day. Maggie suggests:

> Request a different "day of donation" when reordering sperm. It was explained to me that when sperm is donated to a sperm bank, the sample is split up into several (four or five) tubes. Only one tube is used per IUI. Therefore, if a guy has a bad day (meaning he usually has good quality and quantity sperm) on a given day of donation, then you could possibly get his lower-quality sample in two consecutive IUI tries.

The usual advice to "just" switch donors can be very frustrating. But a fresh start can be one way to take charge of improving your chances.

Even with a "proven" donor, a good specimen, and proof of ovulation, you may wonder about the timing of inseminations. If you're using medication(s) to develop eggs, you certainly want to be sure sperm are there when they need to be. Rose tried twelve IUI cycles, fortunately covered by insurance, before her specialist ordered daily ultrasounds to see if follicles had ruptured. When a four-day delay after the hCG shot was diagnosed, Rose knew why she hadn't gotten pregnant, with all her inseminations done long before that.

You may wish to pay for a second IUI, especially if the first specimen wasn't great. Most medical teams do inseminations twenty-four hours apart, but some will do two IUIs on the same day, one very early and one late in the day, if they're sure they've pinpointed ovulation. Studies generally show improved pregnancy rates with two inseminations,[9] though if the single insemination is at the ideal time, it will be essentially as good as adding a second too early or too late.

Insemination is the wrong term for some people, who need more high-tech procedures—IVF, GIFT, ZIFT, and so on. This is the alphabet soup you probably were hoping to avoid with donor insemination. But these reproductive technologies may be needed because of female infertility. Because Shannon knew about the possible impact of her severe endometriosis on pregnancy rates, she felt that intrauterine insemination attempts were futile. After months of trying, she lamented that "each time we try, it seems we discover new problems we never knew existed." Her doctor agreed that IVF with donor sperm would offer greater chances of beating the odds. Rose, whose response to hCG was so delayed, finally became pregnant in her first DI IVF cycle because her eggs were removed at the ideal time. Blocked tubes or age pressures can lead quickly to ARTs.

Health insurance may pay for IUIs, even for expensive medications, but balk at ARTs. Couples have taken jobs just because of insurance coverage or even moved to states with ART mandates. The cost of ARTs moves many couples toward ending treatment.

Once you're using medications that develop several eggs, ARTs offer advantages over IUI. Removing the eggs from ovarian follicles and bringing them into the laboratory allows analysis of your egg and embryo quality. This is especially important for women over thirty-five and with ovulatory difficulties. Removing eggs, instead of letting them release within the body for IUI, allows the freezing of any "extra" embryos, which can be thawed and transferred in a later cycle without your having to take further egg-developing medications. Frozen sperm also seems to be less impaired when it comes to fertilizing eggs in the embryology laboratory.

If a woman responds poorly to ovulation-inducing drugs, she may make only a few eggs or only poor-quality eggs, no matter how much medication is used. The ovaries often begin to slow down in the decade before menopause, and some women go through premature menopause. For some the most promising option is to also seek out donated eggs. This is often seen as going too far for a pregnancy because neither parent will share genes with their child. Those who try "donor/donor" or "DI/DE" cycles often have a strong longing to be pregnant or strong reservations about adopting. You'll want to seek out added information on this newer alternative.

Other couples reaching the stage of discussing assisted reproductive technology options wonder whether to continue using donor sperm or to try these advanced techniques with the husband's sperm. If they're going to face the stresses of IVF, they may now find themselves considering intracytoplasmic sperm injection (ICSI) with the husband's sperm. IVF laboratories can "micromanipulate" eggs and sperm to increase the chances of embryos forming with even a single sperm. Unfortunately, ICSI is expensive, adding more expense to already high IVF costs. After four failed DI cycles, Becki's specialist suggested using IVF with ICSI. As Becki wrote in the midst of her decision making:

> It's such a Catch-22—if we use our savings, there goes the college fund; but if we don't, we won't even need the college fund. My husband is especially leery of spending so much more on what's essentially a crap shoot.

Unless you have insurance coverage for infertility, high-tech efforts, with husband or donor sperm, may be financially impractical, stressful, and quite brief.

It's important that spouses help each other avoid becoming overly focused on medical success. You can go off on a quest for the "right" answers or the "best" expert. But at some point you may find it more rewarding to focus on your well-being and on the options that lie ahead.

WHAT ALLOWS YOU TO CONTINUE?

Continuing to try can lead to one of two possible good outcomes. The obviously preferred success is the pregnancy you've worked so hard for. The other success is a stronger sense that you did all you reasonably could and that you've used this time to begin grieving and moving toward other alternatives. You may have read about "resolution" in some infertility books, the stage of the grieving process that RESOLVE's name is based upon. You may fear that you'll never feel resolved if DI doesn't work, that you'll always have regrets, wondering if you did enough. Certainly, many say they didn't begin to feel much better about their decision to end treatment until they were well beyond the Trying Times.

You do need to learn what's reasonable, what's medically warranted if you decide to continue treatment. You may have assumed that DI's quick success would spare you becoming an expert on female fertility or insemination options. It's hard to know when to stop, when to ignore that voice saying, "We've already come this far . . . the next cycle will be it." Parents whose persistence was rewarded later sound amazingly sure it was all worth it. Karen reports in a RESOLVE newsletter:

> Infertility consumed us for three long years and will always be a part of our lives. Every time we look at our daughter we feel it was worth every injection, every side-effect from the medication, the two or three inseminations a month, and every tear. I have one word of advice for couples going through the "trying" to get pregnant stage. Keep trying. There is no greater joy a couple can have than having a child.[10]

Connie agrees:

> When I finally got pregnant, my line was "We were lucky—it only took us two years." And it's tallied in the end as a laparoscopy, a miscarriage, a clinical pregnancy, a hysteroscopy, two HSG X-rays, six vaginal inseminations with no drugs, six IUI inseminations, two with drugs for the first pregnancy, and two with drugs for the second pregnancy, and two years of progesterone suppositories. I can't believe that it was my life! But we have a healthy son to show for it.

But many tryers can't wait much longer; they're becoming too broke, too stressed, or too disillusioned. If you or your spouse is starting to have doubts about continuing, it's important to think about how you'll decide when to stop, how you'll know when you've done all you should. With all the medical options available, it's unlikely you'll be told by your doctor to quit. You need to keep an eye on the other DI costs, not only the medical bills but also those that drain your emotional and marital resources. It's important to have some sense of limits, even if they're only loose guidelines, not strict rules. Ready for her final attempts, Peggy, trying on her own, writes:

> I'm planning to do two more GIFT cycles. I can handle it physically and financially, but I don't know about the emotional fallout from further loss. With the help of my counselor, therapist, and RESOLVE, I'm considering family building through adoption.

Having a pregnancy, becoming a parent, is an incredibly important goal, but it can't be accomplished at the expense of your health, relationship, job, or financial stability. If these are being seriously endangered, take a break and allow some time off for healing, for considering if you can continue in this direction. Sarah explains:

> I was tired of trying and paying out so much money every month. So . . . I decided to take a break and it's the best thing I could've done for my

psyche. I'm back to eating healthy, exercising every day, and just getting back in touch with me and my life with Andy. I'm happy and relaxed!

If you decide to continue with DI, you may fear becoming a medical information junkie. Many jokingly say they could teach reproductive endocrinology. You need to be obsessed enough to keep track of details, observations, and questions for your medical team. Learning to manage the Trying Times, being aware of ways to maximize each cycle, cutting costs, and reducing your stress and effort may allow you to continue longer than you might have expected. A couple discussion after each cycle can help you review what you learned from the last and what you need to anticipate in the decisions ahead.

It's important to acknowledge the emotions that failed cycles stir up. Peggy remembers:

> The biggest loss is the disappointment of not conceiving each cycle and the loss of hopes and dreams. Each cycle I would grieve for my lost eggs, which I considered to be my "babies." When transvaginal GIFT using donor sperm didn't succeed, I felt like my body was failing me. I had just lost five potential babies, and most of all, I felt a loss of my fertility.

There can be silver linings to the black cloud of DIs not working quickly. If you become pregnant after many months, DI doubts will usually have receded. Shelley, who became pregnant only after she and Jim turned to both donated eggs and sperm, explains that "once infertility treatment takes over, the issues around donor choice fade into the background." Anne recalls:

> Each time was a loss that felt as painful as if we'd used Clyde's sperm. There were actually times when we practically forgot about the donor aspect—we were just so disappointed each month when I got my period.

Sooner or later, those who aren't quickly successful begin to wonder what will happen if this option also fails. Some become discouraged early on. Becki writes:

I've just gotten my period, two weeks after our second attempt at DI. To say I'm devastated is a huge understatement. We decided on DI after a year of monthly intrauterine inseminations using my husband's sperm. After a year that was a roller coaster of emotions, I'd convinced myself that this was the answer to our problem. Now I'm devastated to think there may not be an answer.

The pressure on women can escalate quickly. Peggy reports:

A major loss I've experienced is a familiar infertility loss, loss of control. My cycle would control me. My schedule was no longer my own. I wouldn't always know the date, but I always knew what day I was on in my cycle.

Sandy looks back on grueling Trying Times.

To be stubborn, hard-headed, and to withstand physical and emotional pain are probably my recommended prerequisites for DI or any form of infertility treatment . . . what a strange process! My husband supported me all the way: he let me cry and shared my occasional joy. But he, more than I at times, never gave up. I couldn't have made it without him.

When More Bad News Strikes

For some couples the Trying Times are tragic as well. One of the saddest outcomes of a DI cycle is the loss of a pregnancy. Sometimes an early miscarriage offers hope that you've come close to success. But for many, a pregnancy failing is the beginning of the end. Chris's second miscarriage was a turning point:

I really knew this time I'd hit bottom. My vision of the world began to change once again. I understood that I'd better get off this baby chase and take care of myself. . . . I'd come to the realization that the risk of another miscarriage was totally unacceptable to have some "stranger's kid." . . .

Frozen sperm with its lower success rate began to replace fresh sperm as the accepted option. The forces that propelled us toward DI were slowly pulling us away. We made the decision to pursue adoption.

While any couple going through a loss wonders how they could ever try again, couples who have to return to the extensive treatment of DI feel desperately unable to contemplate starting all over. Ann and William's baby was stillborn at twenty-two weeks. Ann remembers:

> One of the things that struck so hard was how life could go from the highest of highs to the lowest of lows in the blink of an eye. William and I were so incredibly happy when I was pregnant with Hannah. For the most part, the misery of DI had disappeared with the positive pregnancy test. . . . Then the shock of my life occurred when my water broke, and I knew right at that moment that it was over, this baby would not survive this. How could life be so cruel—twice? And I asked myself, "What have I done to deserve this?" and then I answered that question with a hundred responses. I was so unprepared for these tragedies.
>
> When my next pregnancy, with Alaina, ran into trouble, I was no longer the naive person who said, "It will be all right, it can't happen again" but rather, "I can't believe this is going to happen to me again. This time I won't survive it." . . . Despite some very difficult, anxious moments, however, this pregnancy was also a joyous time for me, and the miracle of Alaina's birth and the precious miracle that she is fills me with emotions that are too difficult to put into words.

Sometimes the tragedy is that the marriage is in serious trouble. One infertility myth is that it always brings a couple closer together. Patricia refers to herself as a "go with the program type," and she assumed she and her first husband shared a total commitment to the priority of having a baby. But he didn't speak up when he began to lose connection with her as well as that program. One night as they began another DI IVF cycle, he announced that he couldn't give her the shot—and that he didn't love her, didn't even want kids. During the shock of their separation, they came to see that they'd intellectually agreed on each step of treatment but hadn't kept up with the overwhelming emotional toll of their high-tech DI attempts. While this marriage did end, many couples can recover if they find the resources to sort out what went wrong and reconnect. Taking a break from treatment can be vital, though agonizing when there's no break from childlessness.

Sometimes the bad news that strikes is unrelated to infertility, but it's just the final straw. If DI cycles happened in a vacuum, with no other stressful things going on, maybe you could indefinitely keep trying, hoping to hit that lucky cycle. But when other crises happen, along with the daily issues of life, many couples begin to realize they're becoming tremendously drained.

WHEN IS ENOUGH ENOUGH?

For some, thinking of their next alternative, a backup plan, is empowering. For others, there is only overwhelming despair triggered by the thought of ending DI attempts. No matter what feelings are stirred up, it's important to set aside some time for occasional talks about "What if . . . ?" It's not wise to talk about this nightly, at least not until you really are close to saying "Enough." But it is important to talk long before you're on the verge of a major conflict over whether to commit to the next level of treatment or end treatment altogether.

The decision about how far to go is unique for each person. It's often said in infertility groups that you'll know when it's time to stop. But it's important to learn all you can about how others have known, because there are common blocks to realizing you've had enough.

One block can be your own personality. Traits that can be so valuable in other situations, where your efforts play a strong role in your success, can work against you here. Stubbornness, determination, optimism, and faith are all examples of qualities that can keep you trying for a pregnancy. If you decide to broaden your goals, to look at reaching for parenthood or happiness some other way, you may be able to redirect yourself toward these new goals.

Some people do have a hard time letting go of their first choice. Ending DI might make you feel like a two-time loser, but perhaps you could redefine emotional resolution as your goal, acknowledge that happiness was what you always wanted. If your goal isn't just pregnancy and medical success, you're more likely to stop to consider if DI still seems like the best pathway to happiness. Depression, aggravated by Clomid, was the stopping point for June.

> I knew that I couldn't do any more, and Alan knew he didn't want to either. So then I really got depressed because I knew we'd never have the pregnancy I'd dreamt of for so many years. Grieving is the pits, but it sure has taught us a lot. So here we are headed toward resolving in our own way. It still hurts now and then, but the last two months are the first I have not cried myself to sleep when I start my period. . . . Alan and I are midway in adopting a baby from China.

Deciding you've had enough is difficult for couples because it's unusual to come to that point at the same time or for the same reason. Why one of you might want to continue with DI will have a lot to do with why you chose DI in the first place. John, who had to confront adoption when Chris couldn't imagine facing another DI miscarriage, had chosen DI because it could be so private. As he considered ending treatment, he still dreaded the invasion of a home study and everyone knowing they "had" to adopt. (Ironically, he's now done public speaking on adoption.) It's difficult to accept that you're at the point of considering ending treatment because your spouse is.

Stopping DI is usually more difficult for women than for men. Men have already been adjusting to the idea of parenting a child not biologically related to them. And seldom is the childbirth experience as compelling a longing for men as it is for women. Erin writes:

> It is, I think, easier for the male who has the sterility problem to feel more detached . . . he doesn't have to go through all the medical trials

and tribulations. For him the question of fertility is over. For the female partner it is a constant. The male (in our case) is just glad to be alive, free of cancer. Kids are icing on the cake. . . .

I think part of the reason adoption is so appealing is that it takes the situation and turns it into a positive one. Adoption will work. There are no bodies involved. There is no sense of "Why is this failing?" One can have sex again without wondering why such a normal act doesn't produce a normal event. . . . My goal is to be a parent. I would love to be pregnant, but my real goal is to be a parent. I grieve not seeing Sam's great legs in our child or other family traits. But I won't let this stop me from becoming a parent.

Women giving up on DI face the end of their genetic continuity for the first time, as well as the loss of connection to other women who have experienced pregnancy and childbirth. Men may assess rationally that adoption offers the certainty of a child or that accepting childlessness will end a project that's been a drain on the couple's life together. Many men speak of being angry at their wife's persistence, at her refusal to look at the costs of continuing DI. This is a time when many couples seek out counseling because they're at such different places that they can't objectively help each other through the stage ahead.

Many couples feel terribly stressed over money at this stage. And many feel ashamed that money could play a big role in such a profoundly emotional and spiritual decision. You can't afford to go bankrupt. However, you can't spare yourselves expense, and later find you're emotionally or maritally bankrupt because childlessness was cheap fiscally but not a good choice for the two of you. Sometimes you need to take a break to rebuild financial resources as you reframe your family-building plan.

Some people know it's time to stop when it's time for high-tech DI. Many couples who tried insemination with the husband's sperm before undertaking DI stopped short of ARTs during that process, and decide to set that limit again. Wendy allowed herself very limited exposure to fertility drugs because she was trying for a DI pregnancy,

just as worries surfaced about links with ovarian cancer. Since she'd
lost her mother and aunt to this disease, she felt it would be crazy to
persist with ARTs when she was already at too high a risk for cancer.
It was difficult to leave DI behind when she'd been so actively involved
in a group of couples planning for openness, but adoption proved just
as joyous a pathway to parenthood.

In the face of the many feelings stirred up by ending treatment, it
may be hard to view any alternative positively. Aline Zoldbrod, in
Getting Around the Boulder in the Road, recommends:

> If you find yourselves nearing the point of ending the quest for a biologi-
> cal child, conscientiously practice creating vivid, positive images about
> parenting an adopted child, or about childfree living. What will your life
> look like? What is there to look forward to? What will you do together?
> Make your images as concrete as possible. IF YOU CANNOT COME
> UP WITH ANY POSITIVE IMAGERY, YOU SHOULD GET SOME
> PROFESSIONAL HELP.[11]

DIFFERENT DREAMS CAN COME TRUE

There comes a point when you need to envision a new resolution. You
don't want to hear anyone suggest this will be easy, as in platitudes like
"There are so many kids to adopt!" or "Ann Landers did this study
that showed couples without kids really are happier!" Ending your
hopes for a DI pregnancy may prove almost as difficult as your initial
grieving after the loss of hope for a genetically shared pregnancy. But
you may be surprised to feel some relief too, especially if you've been
trying for a long time or with great difficulty.

Adoption is a wonderful way to create a family, a truth as often
overlooked as it is for DI. No, the process and the payments aren't
usually fun. As with DI, there will be lifelong challenges, whether for
yourself or for your child, whom you want so much to protect from
pain. But the sense of the miraculous, the joy in new beginnings, is

just as precious. June writes about completing their home study to adopt from China.

> The process just swept us up as we got into it. I'm surprised and pleased that it feels as exciting as I had imagined only a pregnancy could feel. I actually bought two pink baby booties—having hope again feels so good.

Almost all adoptive parents voice a wish that they hadn't waited so long to adopt—even as they add that they're glad they weren't ready any sooner because then their wonderful child would not have become theirs.

Some people find they can begin to move toward adoption while still trying for a pregnancy, while others need to come to closure on DI before moving toward adoption. Diana's first cycle ended in miscarriage at eight weeks; six more months of trying was enough to add adoption planning to the mix.

> We took the "take-no-prisoners" approach, applying to an adoption agency, taking classes on private adoption, and entering a formal infertility program. . . . After seven more cycles, I told my infertility specialist I couldn't do any more. The Clomid didn't seem to be working. I was emotionally bankrupt, and GIFT, ZIFT, or IVF would have finished us off financially. He accused me of not being committed enough. I noticed his tan. He said he had just returned from the U.S. Open.
>
> We focused on the adoption, and in January of 1992, three years after we began our quest for a baby, we rushed to a hospital delivery room to see the birth of our beautiful healthy daughter.

Anne needed recovery time from treatment before she and Clyde could begin adopting.

> When the last cycle failed, probably because my egg quality was poor, we began our grieving and recovery process. . . . I felt extremely OLD! I experienced sadness I never knew was possible. We took about six months to "heal," though I truly believe that infertility will always be a part of the people we have become, and I'm afraid a part of me will remain with the

unsuccessful pregnancy attempts. . . . In looking back, I feel I stayed in treatment too long and emotionally lost more than I had bargained for.

When you haven't yet adopted, it can be hard to believe you could find the strength to start down this new path. You may indeed have to ask for help, and this is where the greater openness and acceptance of adoption can help. While you may not have kept your family or friends informed about your infertility procedures, you may feel more able to tell them about adoption. Clyde and Anne flew to Siberia to meet their son. Speaking at adoption workshops, they have unexpectedly begun a new commitment, to the world of adoption, helping others begin their families with a visit to an orphanage.

Brian and Tracy also spoke at an adoption workshop, sharing their memories of DI treatment as well as the miraculous open adoption of their son. With each cycle, while learning their last donor wasn't available, they would also discover some new problem with Tracy's fertility. As months passed, they became less interested in pregnancy but definitely wanted kids. One day an old friend called, asking if they were still trying, because her children's baby-sitter was pregnant and considering an adoption plan for her baby. Tracy and Brian began a wonderful process that led them to the delivery room, coaching as their baby was born. They don't feel this was any less miraculous than giving birth themselves.

Those who choose to resolve without children often feel overlooked. It's harder to affirm what society often views as a negative choice, choosing not to adopt. There's often little sympathy for those who realize giving birth was an irreplaceable part of their dream. Unfortunately, some who have resolved to move on in life without children report losing their infertility friends. Those who give birth may avoid your pain or the differences in your lives. Those adopting may assume you have negative feelings about adoption.

Once you've made some progress toward creating your own positive vision of childlessness, you may be ready to share that with family and friends. You may need to teach them, over time, to accept that your family-building saga won't end with a baby. This alternative may be far from your first choice, but resolving to live as a family of two can offer a pathway to future happiness for many couples.[12]

When you move on from DI without medical success, it may take years to make peace with this new loss. Feel your feelings, find a way to channel them, and try not to let them harden into bitterness that you ever let yourself try DI. We hope Liza's words hold some truth for you.

> I want to acknowledge what I've gained by becoming infertile and pursuing DI. . . . I'm not ready to sing praises to the benefits of suffering and loss, but it's true that I've had to grow because of infertility. My consciousness has been raised (not unlike going from being able-bodied to being disabled). I feel I'm more mature, stronger in the face of life's challenges, and have a greater capacity for empathy and tolerance.

Chapter Six

Becoming Pregnant:
Shock, Relief, Fear, and Joy

It was our seventh month of trying donor insemination, and we were losing hope that this would ever work. It had become a sad routine. I'd go to the doctor's office for a pregnancy test two days before my period was due. After getting the negative results, I'd cry for the next two days while I waited for my period. Bob had just been through surgery for testicular cancer, and I felt nothing would ever go right in our lives again.

That month's routine was even worse—when I finally got up the courage to call for my results, no one was picking up the phone at the doctor's office. I finally called the sperm bank next door to find out what the problem was. She put me on hold for ten minutes, then told me I could only get my results from the doctor's office directly and their phones were broken. I just started to cry out of frustration, thinking, "Just give me the bad news and let me move on." I guess she felt bad for me, because she blurted out, "You're pregnant." Just recalling that magical moment still brings tears to my eyes.

I wanted to tell Bob in a special way, but by time I got home I was too hysterical to speak. Bob just took me into his arms as he did every month and said, "Don't worry; we'll try again next month." Finally I choked out, "I'm pregnant," and together we cried in joy. Next Bob took out the video camera and started a nine-month documentary of our pregnancy.

For us the nine months were a wonderful time of dreaming and sharing together. For most of our family and closest friends it was a time of adjustment, since this is when we chose to tell them about using donor sperm. We just couldn't go through all the talk about the baby having Bob's eyes and hair without them knowing the truth. Even their questions and concerns didn't affect our special nine months together. I believe our pregnancy was an extra-special experience because of what we went through together to get there. For most of the pregnancy, how we became pregnant was pushed aside. We just enjoyed watching us both get rounder!

—*Heidi*

Hearing "The test is positive!" is expected to be a thrill, the beginning of celebration. Yet when a pregnancy begins via DI, earlier dreams have been greatly changed by time, losses, anxiety, and concerns about whom to confide in. It's important to acknowledge the complexities that might challenge a DI pregnancy without losing sight of all the positive aspects of this time in your life.

How you feel about your pregnancy will be affected by all the past decisions you've made and experiences you've had. If DI was an easy or obvious choice, pregnancy news is much more joyous than for someone who's been in great pain or ambivalence about DI. Those who have been extremely private about DI often feel a greater sense of isolation than those who have had a strong inner circle of confidants. A couple who chose a donor they feel good about will have less anxiety and fewer questions than a couple who felt unable to participate or limited in their choices of donor. Couples may be in greater shock at the news of a positive pregnancy test if they'd just gotten started and expected to have a few cycles to adjust to the process emotionally. In contrast, couples may be more relieved than overjoyed if they've been trying for many cycles, and more anxious than thrilled if fearing a miscarriage or other tragic news.

The news of a positive pregnancy test marks the beginning of a very long process, with many changes, through each trimester, through childbirth, and through the postpartum adjustments. The news can be emotionally overwhelming. Anne recalls her reactions:

> And then I remember the pregnancy test. The positive one. The one where I was SURE I was going to throw up. The one when my life changed forever and ever, more fundamentally than it ever had before or will again. Laughing, crying, trying to stand up, trying to sit down, dancing around with Larry, hugging, hoping, disbelieving.

Connie remembers panic and second thoughts about the donor they had chosen.

> When I had my first positive pregnancy test (a clinical pregnancy) with one donor we'd chosen, I panicked. He was ugly. The father of this baby was ugly! Oh my God, what had I done? I was going to give birth to some horrible kid. I prayed that I could have another chance to switch donors. My prayers were answered and the next day I got my period. I was so relieved. No one, absolutely no one knew how horrified I was to be pregnant.

Grace writes that her reaction wasn't what she had expected.

> After recovering the ability to feel anything, I was surprised that it wasn't the pure ecstasy that I'd anticipated. It was a weird mixture: disbelief, relief, joy, apprehension, guilt, a blessing, a burden, the sensation of having both a big announcement and a big secret. Mostly disbelief.

It's important to allow the full range of responses when the news of a positive pregnancy test finally arrives. This is news you've longed for, not simply from the time you've been trying, but possibly since you met your spouse. There is also some sadness, however, as this child won't be the one you'd always pictured. Fathers-to-be may wonder if they're as proud as they should be. Mothers-to-be may feel they don't really, fully fit in with pregnant women who haven't faced their challenges.

A new pregnancy can also be a frighteningly uncertain time. You may be all too aware that not all positive pregnancy tests lead to babies. Anxiety, especially about early miscarriage, may overshadow any worries related to DI per se. Leigh assumed the worst when she had pain early on:

> A week later I was at the doctor's office because of very sharp pains I was having on my left side. I thought everything was going to fall apart then. . . . It turned out I had a cyst on my ovary and that it would dissolve after a while.

The harder and longer you had to work to get pregnant, the more anxious you're likely to be. As Ellen Glazer explains in *The Long-Awaited Stork*:

> Prolonged infertility causes people to anticipate loss. It convinces them that their bodies do not work right and it heightens their awareness of what miracles conception, pregnancy, and childbirth really are. . . . For them, a positive pregnancy test brings nine months of fear and anxiety.[1]

Some people are afraid they'll "jinx" this pregnancy, either by letting their hopes get too high or by allowing "negative thinking" about all that might go wrong. It's hard to remain logical when a new pregnancy is precious and could be precarious. Heidi spent much of her first trimester in the bathroom, checking for bleeding. This is why many wait to celebrate until they've seen a heartbeat on ultrasound or the amniocentesis report is normal—or until they're holding a healthy baby in the delivery room.

The first weeks are a time of sorting out your reactions and those of your spouse. Women and men often feel differently about pregnancy and babies. Add in DI, and there's potential for confusion and upset.

Many men report feeling very distant at this stage, almost as if their wife and the medical team are celebrating a pregnancy. Some wonder if it was really a good idea to have unselfishly done this "for my wife," a concern especially strong for men who are starting a second family or for men who were ambivalent about ever having kids, no matter what the route of conception. Some may have secretly been hoping that somehow DI wouldn't work and now have guilt-inducing moments of hoping the pregnancy won't succeed. Powerful emotions may come spilling out in words or show in tense or withdrawn behavior.

Women, too, may be ambivalent about the news of pregnancy. Some worry that the DI decision was reached too quickly or wonder if they're as happy as they should be. As Donna puts it, "Ninety-nine percent of the time I'm thrilled, but 1 percent of the time I am crushed that I'm not carrying Harry's baby."

Another common source of concern is increased curiosity about the donor. Some couples may have been so anxious to get started or so uninformed of their options that they didn't learn everything they could have about their donor. Once pregnancy is a reality, one of you may feel the need to get that information ASAP while the other feels it could be distressing. A compromise can be to wait until the baby is born. Once you've fallen in love with your child, you might read that long profile with less distress.

Becoming pregnant quickly can be challenging for infertile couples. If a wife easily becomes pregnant via DI, he may feel more alone in his infertility, though guilty even mentioning this, knowing they were spared months of DI treatment. On the other hand, if you've been through months or years of trying for a DI pregnancy, celebrating can be tough. You may be too tired, broke, and fearful of bad news to be overjoyed. You may feel guilty to be more relieved than happy—"at least I don't have to go back to the infertility specialist next month."

SETTLING INTO THE REALITY OF YOUR PREGNANCY

Take some time to adjust to being pregnant. Before widely announcing your news, process all that it means for you both. If you two have somewhat different needs, it can be distressing. One of you may need a time of not discussing the donor, while the other longs for an in-depth discussion of how this is similar to and different from a genetically shared pregnancy. One may want to tell the world that you achieved this wonderful miracle, while the other feels a stronger need for privacy. One guideline might be to give extra weight and sensitivity to the needs of the nonbiological parent-to-be—although not to the extent of trampling on the needs of his partner. When you've lost your genetic connection to the next generation, you may feel you deserve the right to process what that means to you in your own way, at your own pace. It can be frightening to put powerful feelings and images into words, even with a spouse. It's important not to judge any reactions as signs that DI was a bad choice.

You'll undoubtedly hit some rocky moments with the reactions of others, especially if they don't know of DI's difficulties. For married couples pregnancy is expected to bring celebration and maybe some teasing. Husbands especially report jokes like "I didn't know you had it in you." Few understand that teasing about "We know what you've been up to" is upsetting when what you've been up to is sperm bank orders! You may be asked what finally worked, and you can only think, "The donor thawed well this time."

It hurts when loved ones unaware of DI celebrate the pregnancy news by focusing on blood ties and genetic affinity. This can be especially difficult for men who get comments about passing on the family name or who belong to families with a strong interest in genealogy, family heritage, and ethnic ties. No matter how carefully you selected a donor, you are adding a new set of genes to your family tree. It can hurt to realize others are so interested in preserving and celebrating the genes you can't pass on.

Ironically, insensitive remarks may also come from your inner circle. One of Heidi and Bob's relatives kept insisting that DI didn't make any difference to him and shouldn't to them. This denial of their feelings felt as hurtful as a negative comment about DI. Many of those who are newly pregnant never dared think this far ahead, to actually having good news to share. So they never really told their inner circle how they'd want the topic of DI treated. The news of a pregnancy makes it suddenly a real issue. If you want people in your inner circle to ask about DI, tell them so, and if you want them not to ask about DI, also tell them. Loving supporters still need a signal from you, as they probably have no personal experience with DI to guide them.

In many ways a DI pregnancy is going to be treated just like any other pregnancy, with the indignities as well as the joys. The transition to being a "regular" obstetrical patient can be a big challenge. Most DI pregnancies begin at one facility that assists with inseminations, but care is then transferred to an obstetrician who might know nothing of your DI experience. Obstetrical practices rotate coverage, so you'll have a whole new cast of characters. Many couples choose not to confide in the obstetrician about DI, feeling it's irrelevant medically. (There are more arguments for telling pediatricians, with whom you can confidentially discuss any questions about genetic factors in your child's development.) If you feel close to your obstetrician or midwife, you may want to disclose DI. A new medical practice certainly can't understand all your emotions about your pregnancy, even if the fact of DI is shared.

For anyone who has been in the care of a fertility specialist for some time, it can be surprising to feel "abandoned" or "rejected." You may have assumed you'd be thrilled to be done with intrusive, time-consuming, schedule-ruining fertility treatments, but you may find it anxiety-arousing to see a doctor just for "routine" checkups. Deborah found it wonderful that her obstetrician was sensitive to infertility and invited her to set up more frequent appointments if that would help her feel more secure.

Of course, not all DI pregnancies are routine. Couples who have become very knowledgeable about fertility treatment know that miscarriage is far from uncommon, so the first trimester is often an anxious time. Decisions about prenatal diagnosis are a concern for those now facing what doctors disconcertingly refer to as "advanced maternal age." Any obstetrical problem may leave you feeling robbed of your fantasies of an easy, blissful pregnancy.

A common source of DI-related pregnancy complications is carrying twins, conceived after medications developed extra eggs. If your first pregnancy test suggests more than one embryo has implanted, and ultrasound shows two or more heartbeats, you know you're in for a more challenging pregnancy. If three or more implant, you're in for discussions of selective reduction and prematurity risks, terrifying even when the medical team rallies to advise you.

Even with a "normal" pregnancy, your concerns about DI don't just go away. Rae writes:

> We've been able to emotionally support each other by keeping the lines of communication open. We share in every experience, feeling the baby move, decorating the nursery, going to Lamaze class, etc. We still talk about the feeling of loss too and try to be sensitive to when the other person is having a "down moment." I don't think that the birth of our baby will eliminate our sense of loss over Bruce's infertility. Again, they are two separate issues. We still get pangs when couples we know have a very easy time at getting pregnant on their own.

You're now obviously committed to this path but don't yet have the joyful reassurance of holding a lovable little person. An anonymous contributor to RESOLVE of New York City's newsletter reports:

> My wife . . . is now over seven months pregnant. . . . There are times when I feel like crying, because I was not the one to make her pregnant. Yet, there is also the joy that comes from watching her stomach grow, from hearing the baby's heartbeat, and from feeling the baby kick . . . each day the pain recedes further and further. . . . I know now that the child is really what counts, not how he or she arrives. I no longer feel that it belongs to another man. It is as much my child, as if it were my own genes that had fertilized the ovum.[2]

Some seem to move very easily through pregnancy, with little or no shadow cast by DI's differences. Rae declares:

> Bruce adores my belly and loves to feel the baby move. He feels very much a part of this pregnancy and is getting a kick out of being the

"father-to-be." When one of his sisters gave him a pair of matching sweatshirts that she'd decorated (one for him and one for the baby), it brought tears to his eyes.

Ellen and Kirk had expected to have issues, but she writes, "Strangely enough, we never thought much about the baby being a product of DI while I was pregnant." Grace thinks back on the later stages of pregnancy: "I felt wonderful, have never been happier in my life. . . . Never, before or since, have I lived a dream come true."

As the months of pregnancy move on, it's amazing to finally believe you're moving into the "Fertile World." In her ninth month Emily writes:

> I still marvel at the reality of my swollen belly and the joy I experience as I prepare the baby's room. I must acknowledge, however, that I'm still deeply scarred by the experience of infertility and I ache for the people I know who are still involved in treatment.

It may be shocking to realize how much you once idealized pregnancy. Now you're learning firsthand that it's often overrated. Changes in your sex life, your energy level, your sleep pattern, your diet—these often happen to men as well as women. Because you expected to be a glowing wife and an adoringly helpful husband, you might think you're adjusting so disappointingly because of DI.

As pregnancy progresses, one theme is finding the right balance for each parent-to-be, in how much you acknowledge the role of DI in your feelings about pregnancy. Do you want or need to look at how you are different from others who are pregnant, or how you are similar? You might benefit from seeking out DI parents who can still remember their complicated feelings during pregnancy. But if you have few DI concerns, you may enjoy blending in with other "regular" parents-to-be.

In the third trimester, concerns with the donor often resurface. People who don't want to be widely open obviously hope the baby looks like them, that no one reacts with "Where did he come from?" This often gets jokingly expressed as hoping "no one mixed up the sperm." Anxieties about the donor's contribution are normal—the most common is that the baby will have a huge nose.

When you haven't yet seen the "results" of your donor choice, when you may wish you could leave the talk of sperm banks far behind, you do have some important decisions to make if you used an anonymous donor. This is the time to be sure your pregnancy has been reported to the bank, and the time to make preliminary decisions about reserving sperm for a future pregnancy. Both tasks often get put off, but there are reasons for getting them done now.

Reporting your pregnancy to the bank is often presumed to be your medical team's task. But it's in the parents' best interest to do this themselves. First, the sooner the maximum number of allowed pregnancies is reported, the sooner all remaining vials are limited to use in sibling pregnancies, which makes your next task of reserving sperm easier. It's in your child's interest to limit the numbers of families conceiving with your donor, so that the possibility of her unknowingly marrying another person conceived by the same donor is as minimal a fear as possible. There are arguments for registering yourselves as parents via this specific donor should any new medical information or questions arise.

Unless you're absolutely certain that you'll never try for another pregnancy, it's also important to reserve additional sperm. Some banks have reduced storage fees for sibling pregnancies if sperm is purchased when a pregnancy is reported. (That's one way to encourage the prompt reporting of pregnancies.) Couples often feel very broke and afraid to put out a thousand or two more when anticipating so many baby expenses. Sometimes they're lulled into thinking their donor will be available months later when they can more easily afford to "stockpile" samples. Sperm banks can inadvertently imply that an "ample" supply means the donor will be available indefinitely. Matthew and Laurie's story of carefully choosing their donor is told in chapter 3. The supply of vials from that donor went from one hundred just before their pregnancy to only five soon after their good news—and they'd used many more than five to get that pregnancy started.

A physician who doesn't work extensively with sperm banks may not emphasize the wisdom of reserving now. Only you can fully realize how sad it would be to have to again pick a donor, again wonder about your child's genetic heritage. In addition, you would have to deal with worrying not only if your second child will look like either of you but whether he'll look like your first child. More important than appearance is the security added to siblings' lives to know they're fully related genetically, which might ease any sense of disconnection from their genetic heritage.

The whole topic of another pregnancy may be painful for many. If a wife is older or has female fertility problems, another pregnancy may seem highly unlikely. It may seem impossible to afford another child. It can be confusing for couples with inconclusive male infertility to make DI plans, since doing so implies that hopes of your next child's conception with your sperm are futile. No matter what your situation, it's difficult to look ahead to a future pregnancy when your first one is so present. But some decisions now can prevent a future crisis. Banks should refund money if your reserved sperm isn't needed by your family and can be made available to others. There may be couples who've been praying for those vials because they hadn't bought enough.

FINALLY, THE BIRTH OF YOUR CHILD

Birth is such a miraculous, overwhelming experience that for many new parents, any DI issues are eclipsed by the powerful emotions evoked by their baby's arrival. There's finally a real person here, not an abstraction of family-building goals or donor selection. You'll be busy getting to know this new person, learning to interpret her cries or love his endearing expressions. Anne observes, "What is striking about reading our journals . . . is how very ordinary the experience is. DI babies are just babies when it comes to the mundane matters of growing and being born, sleeping and eating, crying and laughing."

Now is also the time when you'll have to field comments from friends, family, and even strangers. Other people's responses to your new baby are, of course, affected by whether they know of your choice of DI. Your inner circle of supporters will include sensitive people who will follow your lead, letting you raise the topic of DI if you feel the need. Other, equally caring people may assume that you want them to continue to freely discuss DI because that's always been your style. With the exhaustion of childbirth, with the emotions of postpartum, with the protective love of a newborn, you may prefer to set aside DI's impact for now. You might even state this to certain loved ones so that they can stop anxiously wondering if they should be offering you support specifically about DI.

The harder comments to cope with are usually those made by loved ones who don't know how your pregnancy began. It's generally considered socially appropriate with new parents to focus on resemblance— "Oh, he has your eyes" and "Gee, she looks just like Grandma." It's a powerful reminder that genetic influences are assumed to matter a great deal. It makes the nongenetic parent feel left out, the genetic parent feel confused about her feelings of any pride in appearance, and anyone with an anonymous donor aware of how little they know about the donor's features.

How do you cope with comments from those who don't know of DI? When a casual acquaintance makes a comment, you may find the only challenge is to shift the topic from genetic transmission of features to a topic you're happier to discuss, like how cutely her chin trembles when she cries. But when a loved one unaware of DI makes a heartfelt comment ("She has your father's eyes; I wish he could have lived to see this baby"), you may feel so flooded with emotions that you can't get out the responses you so carefully planned. There can be guilt at concealing this information, no matter how thoughtfully you formed your plans not to be open yet with some loved ones. There may be anxious worries that they notice some difference in your reaction, that they do know you turned to DI. There may be deep sadness that your relationship with them at this powerful life transition is complicated by DI. There may be resentment at their stirring up confusing, powerful feelings.

It's important to have some way to regroup, to get back to the centered place in which you can focus on sharing what you do wish to share—your love for the child, your awareness of a loved one's happiness for you. Some parents find that it helps to know they can later talk or laugh with each other or with a loved one who does know of DI. You may also need to shed a few tears or vent some anger later, because some comments are frustrating reminders that society expects babies to be conceived in the "normal" way. Some couples find that turning to humor can get them back on a positive track, especially with images that made them laugh as they role-played scenes earlier in the pregnancy. Quips such as "She really looks like a Martian to us" or "Don't insult my daughter's nose!" can make everyone laugh, providing relief for your tension. Heidi and Bob always commented that their newborns looked like Ed Koch, then the mayor of New York, nearly bald, with puffy cheeks.

If there is any benefit to others' comments, it's that they force you to sort out your feelings. Some new parents find their ability to handle comments and happily introduce their new family member reassures them that DI will be fine. Others find this stage more of a challenge. For a few it brings a resurgence of feelings that must be worked through.

In the first days and weeks with a newborn, you deserve to focus on the bottom line. You're a family, with the baby you've longed for, even if he didn't come into the world exactly as you'd first expected. As the months and years go by, you can count on having to remind yourself of this less often. Eventually someone will comment on who your child looks like, and it will only later occur to you that such comments used to cause you grief.

Chapter Seven

Growing with DI

We look at our children every day and can't imagine how we could be more blessed or happy. Our son is totally a daddy's boy and tries to be just like Bob. Our daughter tells everyone her daddy is the best and cutest in the world. The love between our children and both of us could not be stronger. Even though donor insemination has become a nonissue in our daily lives, it will always be with us as a family and it comes into our minds at times when we least expect it. This would be true whether we chose to be open or private.

Before we told friends about DI, several funny instances that reminded us of DI brought laughs and a little sadness at the same time. One time I was walking down the street with a biologist friend, behind Bob and our son, who were walking the same way and were similarly dressed but looked nothing alike. Our biologist friend commented on how much Bob and our son looked alike, a perfect example of the power of genetics! I wasn't crushed, I didn't need to correct him, but I did feel a twinge. Later I told Bob and we shared a laugh.

—Heidi

You've had a successful pregnancy, and now you go off and live happily ever after, right? Many DI parents have said it's remarkable how quickly they recovered and how happy they feel as parents. One positive side effect of struggling to have a baby is that you're so appreciative of your child's miraculous presence in your life—even at 2 A.M.! As one new mom puts it:

> We think our son is so special, and I think part of that has come from what we had to go through to have him. We have a lot of friends who seem to get pregnant just by looking at people and really have no care or concern for their children. There is a real, deeper love and appreciation that we have for our son; his arrival is the most thrilling thing that has happened in our lives.

But as you'd expect and might fear, DI isn't forgotten once you have your baby. There are times when new concerns will arise, some of them very painful, some extremely challenging. This isn't because you've made the wrong decision or you're coping badly with DI. While our next chapter will look at specific issues for families whose structure isn't so traditional, all parents share some concerns. We do address parents' needs most directly but also hope to support young people and adults who have learned of their DI conception.

Every Child and Family Is Unique

There is no universal "right" way to handle any parenting challenge and there's certainly no one "appropriate" or "healthy" way to feel. Even ill-advised ways of handling DI difficulties are recoverable. It's important not to become immobilized or panicked by fears of the unknown, such as wondering if your child will always remind you of the donor or how to tell your child about DI. Some guidelines can help you form your own ways of coping as a family over the years ahead.

Accepting differences and welcoming diversity are important concepts for DI families. Sometimes your child's personality and behavior will seem unlike yours. It's important not to view her as like her donor and unconnected to you. She's uniquely herself. At her least charming moments, it may be hard to stay calmly focused on helping her shape her behavior and channel her feelings. Her genetic influences don't determine her, and worrisome behavior, such as selfishness, is developmentally normal for children. Some characteristics such as shyness may be inborn to a degree, but the impact can be eased by your nurture. As the authors of *The Personality Self-Portrait* put it:

> Accept and respect each child's individuality. Recognize that his or her temperament is your child's fundamental inborn style. . . . Objectively identify the child's strengths and vulnerabilities, and support his or her positive qualities and individual nature.[1]

Each stage of your child's development brings different issues. You may feel it's alarmist or distressing to read about future parenting problems, assuming "we'll cross that bridge if and when we come to it." For instance, you may not want to think about the possibility that your child could want to know more about her genetic background than you're able to tell her. If you find reading about parenting issues is starting to overwhelm you, step back and remember any challenges will arise only one day at a time. Every possible one won't crop up in your family, and certainly those that do will present you with many healing moments in the months it takes for a family issue to be worked through. If you find yourself continuing to feel anxious or depressed as you think about your family's ability to handle current or future issues, you deserve some added help now. A healthy outlook now will help to bring you greater confidence and comfort as your family grows.

COPING AS A COUPLE, NO MATTER WHAT ISSUE OR STAGE

You and your spouse can have very different approaches and emotional reactions to DI. Allowing each other to have these differences without trying to make one person "wrong" is a great sign for your future success with DI issues. You need to find that balance and acceptance because your child depends on you to be in good shape, both personally and as a couple.

Now that you are parents, you need to keep communicating about donor insemination as a couple, just as you did while you were considering DI or trying to conceive. Even if you're not expecting to talk with your children about DI, it's important that you two talk over issues as they arise. You can't allow DI to become a toxic secret causing tension in your family. You can't get locked into silence or into lifelong promises about how to feel and behave. When one of you has a concern or worry, you need to raise it.

If silence isn't golden, however, neither is constantly focusing on DI. You'll need to decide what to do if one of you needs to talk a lot more than the other. Using one technique, "The Twenty-Minute Rule,"[2] a couple sets aside focused time to talk about feelings and issues surrounding DI. During that time the quieter spouse agrees to be open to talking, and the more communicative partner agrees to limit discussion to this time period. While twenty minutes is sometimes too little, it's amazing how this "rule" can help couples get to the point, and then get off it.

A journal kept by one or both of you can also help. Many DI challenges require reflection. Powerful emotions, such as fear of distressing your child, or traumatic memories, such as the day you learned DI was your only option for a pregnancy, need to find an outlet. If not put into perspective, they can cloud or overwhelm any talk with a spouse. Opinions—yours, your spouse's, the media's, other people's—need to get hashed out. Writing down your thoughts and feelings can help get the topic out of your head.

Keeping a separate family journal will help in the future, especially with telling your child about his genetic background. It would record your family's story of DI; your child may be helped by reading about your loving concern as you learned to live with your DI decisions. The journal will be proof that your choice of DI was one you thought through. One couple found their journal a great help. Their oldest child was very shy and anxious at the age they had originally planned to tell her. They began to realize they might wait until she was more confident, but then she also might be angry with them for not telling sooner. They saw the journal as a way to explain why they'd waited and to share with her what they wished they could have told her each step along the way.

If you are the spouse less inclined to talk things out, you need to acknowledge that there's nothing wrong with your spouse's greater need to discuss DI. But you also need to know that you don't have to totally meet that need. You two can compromise by picking someone whom you both trust to understand your spouse's need for more time on this topic than feels right for you. You may agree that it's OK to confide in a friend or relative who is respectful of confidentiality, empathic, and willing to listen. You might also want to know that this person would be perceptive enough to notice if your spouse were becoming overly focused on DI. You may find it's worth seeking out another DI parent, who will have experience with a number of the issues you're facing. Chapter 9 helps confidants understand how to offer support sensitive to DI.

But many couples find they need to occasionally turn to someone trained in helping couples communicate. It's unfortunately easy for the quieter spouse to drift toward stonewalling any discussion about DI and for both of you to avoid the topic long enough that it comes to feel like a taboo subject. If you're having a hard time discussing DI's impact, you deserve to get some guidance from someone who can help you learn to talk about it in ways that are comfortable for each of you. A counseling professional is ethically committed to confidentiality, which is important for couples who are concerned about privacy.

Life's Not-So-Little Challenges

Some everyday topics can raise challenges for DI parents. You're not crazy if you've become sensitive to and irritated by society's assumption that all families are genetically related. "Blood is thicker than water." "He's just a chip off the old block." These phrases can hurt, just like the command of your church or temple to "be fruitful and multiply," which assumes everyone can do so in the usual way.

But you need to remember to keep DI in perspective. You can incorrectly blame common childhood phases or normal family problems on DI. Your toddler runs to Mom first because that's the stage he's in, not because he feels a preference for his biological parent. Any father might feel rejected by this behavior, but a DI dad losing perspective may take it more personally, seeing it as a reflection of his lack of genetic connection.

DI is not the most important thing about your family. But at different stages in your family's life, DI will bring added twists to parenting.

When You're New Parents

While all new parents must adjust to being Mom and Dad, DI parents have an added adjustment to the differences in how they're connected genetically to their child. The rest of your world needs to come to see you in your new role, and whether or not DI was a difficult choice for you or pregnancy came easily or you've confided in loved ones, this is a challenging stage.

Most parents report that many DI fears start to fade once the baby is born, partly because you're too busy and tired to worry about them. Maura writes, "Because our lives have changed so drastically with his birth, it's very hard to relate to the sorrow of our infertility experience. For both Thad and me, it's over. (Until we try for another!)" Susan reports:

> The child has the potential to be such a positive force in your life that the exact nature and identity of those microscopic parts unknown will remain, for the most part, microscopic in your mind's eye as time goes on. Let expectation, joy, and day-by-day amazement at the magic of growth take over.

Even though the joy of your child's birth may relieve many fears, it may also be a difficult time, because you'll be so often reminded of

DI. Not a day will go by in the first six months of your child's life when someone won't comment on who she looks like. As your child gets older, comments about her looks will probably become fewer and your reactions less intense.

This is a time of testing how you feel about DI. Your child is so little that you don't have to worry about how he's feeling about his origins; he's just focused on his next feeding or where he can manage to crawl to. So you can talk freely with your spouse or with your inner circle of confidants. Of course, many DI parents joke that this is the time when you can tell your child all about DI! Actually, this is good practice—you get to try out expressing your feelings about DI to that little person without worrying about whether you've found the best time, words, or tone. Heidi told her son about DI when he was just two days old; when friends would ask how she planned to explain DI, she'd say she'd already told him and he didn't seem to have a problem with it.

How do new parents react? The most common feelings are amazement, curiosity, and gratitude. No matter how you came to use DI, you probably feel your child's arrival is a miracle. Many times medical miracles were involved. Any curiosity about the donor, whose genes allowed you to have this miracle child, may feel comfortable and natural once your child is in your arms. You'll feel more at peace if you had support in making your decision and in selecting a donor about whom you feel comfortable. If you feel lingering grief over the experiences that brought you to parenthood via DI, you have the rest of your life to make your peace with your losses while experiencing the joy and relief of adding a child to your life.

As You Live out Disclosure Decisions

Once the early months have passed, most parents only occasionally face questions and comments that bring donor insemination to mind. But when you do, you may have to struggle with the reality of living out your decision about how open or private to be. Samantha writes of the problems she and Paul are facing after moving to a new area:

> We're in the awkward position now of being in a new city, making new friends, some of whom look like they will be "keepers," and having to decide whether/when to tell them. One of my classmates asked flat out if we used a donor and I said the suggestion had been made during our workup but that we hadn't done it. I battle with the desire to be open and honest and the desire to control the rate and timing of disclosure. I hate to lie, but I don't think that we are obligated to answer a question simply because it has been asked.

It's often hardest to become comfortable with a "mixed group" made up of someone who doesn't know about DI making "stupid" comments in front of someone else who does know. This is somewhat easier to manage if you've already discussed with your inner circle of confidants why and how to let comments go. Your inner circle probably easily understands why neighbors have no need to know about DI. But they may need your help practicing how to smoothly accept or deflect your aunt's questions about which relative the baby takes after. There may be some awkwardness or guilt at misleading relatives as you actually have to face the emotional reality of earlier decisions to limit the boundaries of your inner circle. You may not have fully realized how your best friend and you would feel when spending time with other, more casual friends not in the know.

Your confidants need to know how to respond when topics steer toward genetic relatedness. The most common approach seems to be complete avoidance of anything genetic. The inner circle never mentions any resemblance to anyone. This can feel like the emperor's new clothes as everyone skirts this very natural topic. You need to teach your inner circle how you want this area handled and model for them how you think about DI. For example, if you're a dad who likes hearing that your baby looks like your wife, because that was a major plus for you in choosing DI, let your inner circle know that those comparisons aren't hurtful for you. You might want to give those closest to you a copy of this book with your favorite stories highlighted to help them understand your feelings and wishes.

If DI is such a powerful issue for you that you want to control when it's raised, then you may be more troubled by loved ones who feel compelled to show you how comfortable they are discussing it. Seldom do parents hear anything explicitly or intentionally negative, but friends may offer overly solicitous and inappropriate reassurance. Karen tells about her experience with a friend:

> She'd visit me and the baby frequently and would always sincerely say, "Oh, he really looks so much like Marty." She was focusing on DI long after I needed to, and she couldn't seem to get over her certainty that Marty and I needed help feeling this was going to be OK. I wished I'd never told her. She hadn't been sensitive during our infertility, insisting I go to baby showers, for example, and I just ended up letting the relationship drift. Because I'd been open with her, I was afraid to let her know how angry I was, for fear she'd retaliate someday by telling others around town. Now if I needed to discuss some things related to DI, I'd most likely talk with other DI parents. They understand how little DI really matters on a daily basis.

While many parents face only a brief stage of questions or comments, it isn't as easy for parents with more striking appearance differences. Carly remembers:

> We suspect Wesley's mother's best friend, who was always at family gatherings, knew something was up. . . . She constantly pried and commented when our daughter was born into a big brown-eyed family with her big blue eyes. Wesley finally pulled her aside and said, "What are you getting at? Do you think my wife had an affair?" He didn't feel we should tell lots of people, especially one so pushy and gossipy, until we decide whether to tell our daughter.

Steve got much less intrusive questions, and lots of positive comments on his daughters, adorable blue-eyed blondes who look just like his wife. But he, too, acknowledged, "I even get jokes about the milkman! It's lucky I feel fine with DI."

When Questions of Another Child Become Pressing

Feelings about the pros and cons of having a second child are tough for most couples. Many fertile couples let nature make the decision for them with a surprise pregnancy. For almost all DI parents, the diagnoses that brought them to DI rule out happy surprises; there's only happiness after much effort. And for many the time, money, and emotional energy it took to have a first child make it difficult to face a repeat performance.

It's not unusual for couples to have differences in their feelings about having another child, and with DI these feelings can take on added force. If one of you felt pressured to do DI, particularly the husband, it can be upsetting to have your spouse raise the topic again. For some who had hoped DI traumas would fade, trying again forces them to resurface.

DI parents often feel their child needs a sibling also conceived with donor sperm. The donor's genetics might be less of an unresolved mystery if there's a fully related sibling, and there'll be someone to share DI discussions. But secondary infertility can cloud your efforts to have another child.[3] Connie writes:

> I want my son to have a sibling, so we are trying again using the same donor. This year we began the infertile life all over again, with months of tests and insurance battles and then nine months of inseminations using drugs and the doctor telling us to switch the donor for better success. I thought we knew how to do it this time. But now I'm into the infertility depression again. All of my son's friends now have or are expecting siblings. He thinks babies are so cute.
>
> This time my husband wants another baby even more than I do. I guess the first time he hadn't realized how satisfying it would be to come home to a kid who loves you because you're his daddy. He's willing to spend the big bucks this time, put our bodies through even more hell. We believe we may have a chance. But that chance is slight. So I spend my waking hours (like now at 3 A.M.) resolving that we'll have only one child, and being thankful that he's healthy. We're a happy family of three.

The ability to envision happiness as a single-child family is a blessing. If you reach your limit in trying for a second, whether that limit is financial, medical, or emotional, you may hit a wave of grief. It's important to know you can get through that grieving process and live joyously as a family of three.

Some parents are committed to adding another child, even via a different pathway. You may have drawn great comfort from thinking your second child would be a little replica of your first, even if you know genetic transmission doesn't work like that. If you didn't reserve enough frozen sperm and your donor is no longer able to donate, you may feel especially bad about missing that chance for your children to share one genetic heritage. You may not find intracytoplasmic sperm injection (ICSI) with your own sperm that comforting; it may only seem like an emotionally confusing, financially costly long shot. Sal and Barbara turned to donor insemination for their first child because his infertility was untreatable before ICSI was developed. By the time they were ready for a second child, ICSI using a few sperm cells surgically removed from the testes was an option, but a complicated one. After many consultations, they decided to turn again to donor insemination. Some families facing secondary infertility consider ending all medical attempts and adding to their family through adoption. Laney and Adam conceived their first child with the help of his brother. Laney reports on their second Trying Times:

> During the last six months . . . there were more unanswered questions.
> There were seemingly unending 50-minute (each way) trips to the medi-
> cal center for intrauterine insemination or whatever. . . . Trying for a
> second child was a full-time job in itself. Also by now we had a challeng-
> ing three-year-old who began to absorb some of this infertility informa-
> tion. She was surrounded by it. She loved to pretend-play being pregnant
> and giving birth. To my surprise her play included getting pregnant by
> going to a doctor's office to have the sperm put in. We hadn't told her
> that! . . .

It was also the continued secrecy that added to our stress. Many people knew by now that we were using medical intervention in attempting a second pregnancy but didn't know we were using donated sperm, didn't know that our daughter was conceived through DI with a sibling donor. These people were a wonderful support during this infertility process and the adoption process to come, but I wish they could have known more, to understand the depth of the grieving.

When Laney and Adam decided enough was enough, they set aside time to mark closure. "The ritual helped us resolve our grief and loss and move on to another way, another child. A year and a half after this ritual, we had a newborn baby girl through adoption." Our next chapter offers guidance for these "blended" families. No matter how you complete your family, there is relief in being done with the stresses of family building.

When DI Memories Come to Mind

Donor insemination will come up at many unexpected times, but some times are predictable. There will be a number of "anniversary reactions" when something will remind you again of DI—the anniversary of your first having DI recommended, the month of your first cycle using donor sperm or of the pregnancy test that led to your child's birth, the time of year when tragic events, such as a miscarriage, happened. The bad news of a biopsy at Thanksgiving will be remembered in future holiday seasons. Your child's birthday may bring thoughts of that special gift from the donor. Some people actually remember dates; others remember a season. Michelle writes:

> Sean had bought me a pot of daffodils the day I went into labor, during a February thaw. When I came home from the hospital, the buds had all opened. We used to say a prayer for the donor, thanking him, on James's birthday, but now I think of him more whenever we have an early thaw, a warm winter day, and whenever the daffodils bloom.

The times in the year that bring back DI memories may at first be a struggle. But as the years go by, any pain associated with those memories fades. And you'll add new memories, of your child's first steps, first day of school, and first date.

It may be challenging when the donor's role comes to mind. When your child develops pride in his talents, some of which mirror those on the donor's profile, it can be confusing. Doing a family tree for school or comparing who in the family has a special talent, a simple task for many families, can bring added challenges for DI parents. When your adult child, starting her own family, wants to talk over her genetic history, you may feel overwhelmed. How you deal with these issues will depend on your disclosure decision, but they do require you to draw on a capacity to think well about DI. You'll need to acknowledge the donor's genetic contribution to your child's life without dwelling on the losses brought by his anonymity or by your loss of shared genetic connection. Focusing on your child's unique personality will help you see her as an individual rather than the product of a donor's genes.

There will be times in family life that hurt, maybe far more so because of DI and more so for fathers: when your child says she hates you; when you feel you're in a devastating power struggle over discipline or your spouse is undermining you with your child in order to look like the nice one; when your child wants to get distance from you, whether at age thirteen pretending not to see you at the mall or at twenty-six deciding to move away for a job. You may wonder how it might have been different if you were all genetically related, if your family were more "normal." Would your child have more difficulty leaving you—or is your difficulty letting him go excessive? At these times you'll have to look to biologically related families to see if they're going through the same things and handling them just as badly as you think you are. Fortunately, these times are the exception, not the rule.

Painful DI issues arise if your child is challenged in some way, not only with more serious issues such as a learning disorder but also if she's just not terribly attractive or socially confident. You may wonder if your child would have these problems if she were not the product of DI—or if you hadn't done DI wrong. Dads sometimes blame their wives, since his genes couldn't be responsible, or both may blame the donor or the bank. It's important to recognize these feelings and talk them through.

As your child grows, gender may play a role in how you feel about DI. Freud may no longer be in fashion, but young sons do have Oedipal feelings for moms and rivalry with dads. Sean and Marty were at a DI parents' meeting, comparing feelings about sons and daughters. Sean reports:

> Marty was saying how his son would actually push him out of bed, saying he was going to marry his mom. I remember that stage; my son would tell me, "I hate you, I wish you weren't my dad." If only he knew, the little monster! Then he came out of that stage and into the "no girls, boys only" stage, when only he, I, and the male dog could go on walks. I must admit I liked that stage much better, but I tried not to play on it too much.

Many men considering DI have said they're afraid to have a son. They worry they'll be even more disappointed if he isn't a chip off the old block or that others will make more comparisons, since sons are supposed to look like their dad, girls like their mom. But, in fact, for DI dads the shared bonds of gender may later come to feel very powerful with a son. With daughters dads need to avoid overrelying on adoration from a "daddy's girl," who will later need to test her independence without your reacting to a resurgence of DI-related fears of disconnection from her. Whether you're the "in" parent or the "out" parent at any particular stage, these issues have little or nothing to do with DI.

As time goes on, it may become easier to accept that reminders of DI are inevitable. While your thoughts and feelings can sometimes be challenging, they don't need to cast a shadow over family life. Rae writes:

> Initially, there was a great sense of loss of our biological child. We still both feel that loss, especially when we see a strong family resemblance

between any father and child. However, we have always separated those feeling from the feelings of joy, love, and excitement about our DI baby. We have found that they're two separate issues for us. We feel so lucky to be able to have a pregnancy and go through the birth of our miracle. This child is still 100 percent our child.

TALKING TO CHILDREN ABOUT DI

Talking with children about DI is a topic deserving its own book, but here we can give you the basics, providing a foundation for decisions about discussing DI as a family. We hope to help you develop the confidence and calm demonstrated by a dad writing to RESOLVE members.

> I love my children, and why shouldn't I? They interact with me just as any children interact with any father. They look at me when they need help, when they want to play, when they want to be affectionate and even when they want to be obstinate. My children don't ask me for family traits; they ask me for attention and caring, hugging and loving.
>
> I'm certain that some day they will ask me "Where did I get my blue eyes, Daddy?" and I will have to tell them that biologically they aren't mine. I don't know how they will react. I can just hope that they will be able to handle the answer. I suspect they will go through periods of being hurt, confused and possibly isolated by it all. And that will be the true test of my fatherhood. If I have properly taught them to appreciate life the way I have, I suspect they will make it through their difficulties.[4]

There are no magic words, no formula that will work for everyone. You're starting a dialog that you want to be open-ended, guided by your child's needs, not controlled or cut off by yours. You'll need to feel comfortable with DI yourself before parent-child discussions begin. You'll need to remember you made the best decision for your family even when your children are struggling through issues that come with DI.

One major concern for parents is protecting their children. Tom Riordan, a dad through both DI and adoption, explains:

> We expect that our son will go through times when he is troubled by DI, just as our daughter will be troubled at times by her adoption and other normal children will be troubled at times by their ethnicity, religion, or some part of their anatomy. "If only I wasn't . . ." and fill in the blank. This is a common child's entry into fantasy escape.[5]

It's difficult to allow your child to have her feelings and work them through in her own way. You won't be any more perfect at this than at any other heroic parental task. You'll most likely underreact or overreact, at least briefly. And your child will recover, more easily if you can make it clear that everyone in the family will be able to grieve losses and grow from this. You can help each other face any insensitivity or ignorance. Tom explains:

> One day someone who really wants to hurl a barb at him will say something hurtful about DI, instead of some other insult. . . . "Your father was a test tube!" And I'm sure it will zing. But neither Joanna nor I are foolish enough to think that we can protect our kids from ever being zung. What we can do is prepare them for life's zings and arrows by helping them develop clear and strong self-images.

Another concern is how children will react to their father once they know. For many couples this is a painful issue as moms watch dads become fearful or reluctant to talk of DI, even when there has been a long-standing agreement to talk as a family. Leigh writes:

> I had always planned on telling them where they came from. . . . Gary also started off that way, but now that he has such a loving relationship with the children, he's very, very frightened about how telling them will affect their relationship.

Ellen reports:

> I began to feel Sophie had the right to meet her biological father, at least
> after she turned eighteen. Kirk was very threatened by my saying I felt this
> way and for a while felt that wanting this devalued his contribution to
> parenting Sophie. He said his biggest fear was that she'd meet her biologi-
> cal father, prefer him, and not want anything else to do with him after that.

It's tough to trust that your child's love and admiration have nothing
to do with shared genetic heritage. If you pull back in fear and miss
out on shared love and fun, you might think DI was the problem when
in fact your protective distancing was.

If and when you choose to talk to your children about DI, it's
important to present a positive image and to give them information
appropriate for their developmental stage. Unfortunately, even the
experts disagree on ideal timing—some advocate early telling,[6] while
others believe DI can't be understood until ages eight to ten.[7] Aline
Zoldbrod, author of *Men, Women and Infertility*, helps her clients imagine how they'll answer crucial questions at each stage.[8] The easy
beginning explanations given to an unquestioning three-year-old will
not present the painful difficulties of answering the questions of a teen
or young adult. Ronny Diamond, a family therapist specializing in
infertility and adoption, reminds parents to move slowly in filling in
all the details.

> Although it is crucial not to lie to your child and pretend you don't know
> things that you know, it is equally crucial to talk with children about
> issues they are developmentally ready to hear. A parent can say, "That's
> an important question, but it's a little too complicated for you to under-
> stand at this age. As you get older I guarantee we'll talk about it more."[9]

Anne Bernstein, author of *Flight of the Stork*, offers excellent advice for
parents as she explains the developmental stages children go through
in understanding sex and reproduction, concepts that underlie a fuller

understanding of DI.[10] Lois Melina's *Making Sense of Adoption* looks at talking with children about DI as "semi-adoption." Reading books and articles may help you find confidence as you find your own way to talk with your child.

As a child becomes aware of the meaning of DI, you can expect questions about the donor. You may or may not have answers to give, depending on how much information you received about the donor years before. Jim and Shelley went to a sperm bank with identity release, believing this would make it easier to handle their son's questions about the donor.

> We know that we can't know all the answers ahead of time! We also know we share a commitment to helping him trust his own understanding of who he is by answering questions forthrightly with sensitivity toward his developmental level of understanding. Slowly from time to time he'll want to understand more. How much more? We have no way of knowing.

Answering questions raises different issues if you know your donor. There will be an actual person with whom the child may well have a good deal of contact, who may be a beloved uncle or dad's old friend, and the questions will obviously be affected by the family's relationship with the donor. Ann and Larry asked a longtime friend to be the donor; he's now an important part of their family life, "Papa John."

> There will likely be times in her life when she will treat this information in a matter-of-fact way and other times when she'll abhor the thought that she's different. So far she knows that she has a Papa John whom she loves to see.

How do you tell a child about a donor if you know almost nothing? You could tell your child about the "typical" donor. Your child's thinking about the donor may be guided by what is statistically likely: the donor was probably open-minded, willing to deal with societal controversies over DI, maybe even enjoying being a bit different or daring; he had a good health history and was intelligent; he was confident enough about himself and his heritage to call for an interview with a sperm bank. This must all be adapted to your child's level, from the preschool explanation of "a nice man helped" to an adult-to-adult sharing of research articles on donor characteristics and motivations.

With or without much information, parents wonder how their child will attempt to relate to his biological father. Just as you mourned the loss of creating a child through sharing your genes, your child will mourn the loss of social connection to his genetic parent and the loss of genetic connection to his dad. It's important that children have nurturing, supportive parents who can accept feelings of confusion, anger, or sadness.

Talking to other DI parents can be invaluable in helping you prepare to talk to your child and in helping you to deal with the results. So you may need to devote time and long-distance phone bills to tracking down others who have also been through this process.

When Your Child Is a Toddler

Many parents and professionals believe that you should begin introducing your children to DI as early as possible. If early telling feels best for your family, you'll need to become knowledgeable about the perceptions of young children.[11] Articles and books on parenting after infertility offer advice:

> DON'T MIX CONCEPTION AND BIRTH. Children under age 3 may not be able to grasp the birds and the bees, but they can appreciate the events of their birth. Stress how excited everyone was about your child's arrival and how you spread the news. . . .
>
> REASSURE YOUR CHILD SHE'S THE SAME AS OTHER KIDS. Before you rush to explain special arrangements or exotic medical techniques, be sure to tell your child, "All babies are made with a sperm and an egg" and "All babies grow in a woman's uterus."[12]

Books such as *How I Began* were intended to help parents talk with very young children. Sometimes the skill is learning that more is not better, that you don't have to spill out everything at once. Genetics is a pretty complex topic, better reserved for later stages. This is also too soon for your child to fully understand your sadness in whatever brought you to DI, although he may watch you facing the stress of more DI treatment for a hoped-for sibling.

The language you use will be taken quite literally at this stage. For example, the imagery of seeds interests young children, and you might explain you had no seeds to grow babies, so you went to the doctor who helped you find a nice man with lots of seeds. Elizabeth Noble recalls using this image with her daughter, then three.

> Julia . . . was much more concerned with understanding why the seeds were absent. . . . The theme was followed up in the vegetable garden, when we observed infertile seeds that she helped to plant and which did not come up.[13]

But don't be surprised if gardening, doctors, and babies all trigger excited retellings of the very special story of her beginnings. Grace is one parent who has begun to put her belief in early telling into practice.

> I never wanted there to be any memory of being told, of not knowing and then knowing. We felt strongly that we wanted her always to know. So since her birth we have spoken openly about "the donor." She loves music, and watching her dance I might remark that the donor loved music too, that he was a music teacher. . . . We compliment the lovely curls in her long hair and comment that the donor had curly hair too.

Young children love to hear stories about their own beginnings. You can use children's books on family-building alternatives as models for your own storybook of your child's beginnings, a longtime technique in adoption. Grace incorporates the story of her daughter's conception in a bedtime story.

> Once upon a time there was a mommy and a daddy who wanted to have a baby of their own. And they waited and they waited for a long, long

time, but no baby ever came. So they went to the doctor, and they found out that a little part inside of the daddy's body, the part that makes the special cells that make babies, was broken. It didn't work right, and they wouldn't be able to make a baby together. But there was another man, a man that they never did meet. This man was called the donor. That part of his body was not broken, and he made it so that the mommy and the daddy could use the special cells from his body to have a baby.

They went to the doctor and the doctor put the special cells from the donor into the mommy, and then a baby started to grow in her tummy! And her tummy got bigger and bigger, and they could feel the baby in there, and they loved her very much. The mommy and the daddy were so happy because finally they'd have a baby to love. And they never got to meet the donor but they were happy and grateful to him because he helped them to make this beautiful baby.

And then everyone was very happy. And they called her Evy, and they loved her so much. And the baby was you! It was you all the time, in the mommy's tummy! But they didn't know that it was Evy until she came out of the mommy's tummy, and now she is such a big girl . . . and her mommy and daddy love her so much.

Grace says that she hated the way the word *sperm* jolted the sentences, so she called them *special cells*. She admits, "I know that still she has no clue, but I feel like I'm laying the foundation for (I hope) easy acceptance. . . . Who knows?"

Should you choose to tell your toddler about his origins, don't expect to get too far before he loses interest. "A nice man helped us have you" may be as far as you get. Anne writes:

I started telling her the story of her creation almost as soon as she was born. Shortly after she was born, I wrote the story down but managed to avoid illustrating it for two years. For her second birthday, I finished the story. To my surprise, she's not all that interested in the storybook (there are very few pictures of her in it!), but writing the story was good practice for telling it to her out loud in the future.

Over time, even young children incorporate your information into an understanding of DI. Joanne tells of the first time the topic of DI was relevant to a question Ray was curious about.

> From the beginning we were committed to telling Ray about his origins "early and often" so at three years of age when friends of his were about to have a new sibling and he wanted to know how babies are made, I began the process. I began by saying, "There are two ways . . ." and I explained DI and intercourse in very simple and concrete terms. Certainly this was an oversimplification (these days there are far more than two ways!), but I think this was enough for a three-year-old's understanding and I wanted from the start to convey a sense of normalcy about his beginnings. What is not clear to me is how often we should be adding to his understanding of DI in light of his maturing understanding of the world. Should we wait until he asks more? Should we initiate from time to time? Given my questions, it was reassuring to see Ray treat the subject of DI in a very accepting, matter-of-fact way in the following exchange when he was five. He asked me, "Mom, what color are your eyes?" "Green." "What color are Dad's eyes?" "Hazel, kind of a gray-blue." "Oh, so green and hazel make blue because my eyes are blue." "Well, genes work differently from mixing colors, but do you remember what we told you about Daddy not having enough sperm to make a baby?" "Oh, so the one whose sperm it was had blue eyes." "I don't remember. Let me check a paper I have about that." (I went and checked the donor sheet.) "Hey, guess what? His eyes were hazel like Dad's and his hair was light sandy brown like yours. Do you have any other questions you want me to answer?" I took a very deep breath as he paused for what seemed like a very long time. "Yes, did this extension cord come with the new fan?"

There are certainly more opportunities for a first child to learn about DI if you're trying for a second pregnancy when they're three or four. Samantha reports:

> We have a number of books for DI kids, and we read them to our son every so often. He knows that the doctor helped us get a seed from

another man because Daddy's seeds weren't working, but he hasn't asked much more than that. We talk about how we wanted him for so long . . . and he knows that children join families in different ways. This is somewhat easier to talk about with him because when I was in treatment to conceive my other son, he came with me to a couple of appointments. He saw the microscope screen with the sperm on it (the doctor told him they were "fish"), and he was right there when the doctor inseminated me. I actually think that he thinks that when people want a baby, they make an appointment with the doctor!

Even young children can sense that something's up, especially if treatment again becomes rigorous or prolonged. One four-year-old was used to the monthly routine when his parents were giving husband insemination another try. Daddy would come out of the bedroom with a brown paper bag and he and Mommy would get in the car to go to the doctor's. The month his parents started DI again, this perceptive little boy helpfully pointed out as they were leaving, "Hey, Daddy, you forgot your paper bag!" He didn't miss a trick.

If you're not planning early disclosure of donor insemination, don't get flustered—he really isn't yet aware of DI. But children are aware of a parent's paranoia, irritation, anxiety, or withdrawal. Even just the sadness or frustration of being back in medical treatment can be detected by young children. You can explain that some people need extra help from the doctor and you're sad because it takes time. He needs to know it's not his fault and not his responsibility to cheer you up, that you'll be OK, and that you have caring grown-ups to support you.

Much more important than sex education is laying the groundwork for self-confidence and for comfort with diversity. Your child can understand that families are formed from love and have many different types of genetic and nongenetic ties. Any children's books that include DI may not be perfectly worded for your family, but they'll get talks started. Taking your preschooler to any activities that make some of this real, such as the holiday party for the program where you became pregnant, may help her get the basics, that some special steps were needed to get her growing in her mommy's uterus. You can mention when someone she knows is part of an adoptive family or a stepfamily so that she will come gradually to realize DI is just one other way to create a family of people who love each other. Children's self-confidence can also grow with the awareness of how much they were wanted. Heidi and Bob's little girl told even the young man filling her McDonald's order that "Mommy and Daddy are very lucky to have me and my brother. Did you know that?"

When Your Child Heads off to School

Once in school, your child's social involvement with playmates and with other adults becomes much more important. And your child can express himself in words, a lot! This stage has some different challenges for wide-open parents than it does for confidential parents or those planning on disclosure at a later stage. The decision to talk with your child requires you to be ready for your family to be more widely open. If your kindergartner has heard positively of his conception, he may of course repeat your story or some garbled version thereof, and you'll have little ability to predict what will trigger his recitation. That can be a scary prospect in a world with even a few judgmental, cruel, or gossipy people.

Children in this age group who have already learned the basics of DI still like hearing "their" story again. As Troy puts it:

> My daughter is thrilled every time I tell her the part about how Mama and Papa were so sad not to be making a baby and how happy we were when the sperm that Papa and the nurse put in Mama's body grew into a baby.

Once your child knows about DI, you'll spend time clarifying confusion. Linda was putting eight-year-old Kate to bed when she asked her mother what was the best thing that ever happened to her. Linda said, "The best thing was when you and your brother were born." Kate replied, "Oh yeah, just me, you, and that guy were there." To Linda's surprise her daughter thought the donor was there at her birth! Linda explained that Daddy was there and the donor is someone they never met. Children may not want details about their donor, but a positive view of him as a helpful or caring person is ideal.[14]

This is the stage when a child can become more aware of any tensions within her more confidential family. She might sense issues in how the adults around her deal with her connections within the family, to Mom, Dad, grandparents, siblings, and others. This tension is what family therapists worry about when DI is an anxiety-producing secret the adults haven't made their peace with. The job for all parents is a continuation of the commitment you made when you decided upon DI—that you wouldn't let your feelings about DI build up or affect your child. This may be the first stage at which you begin to realize fully how adept your child is at reading you, how socially brilliant children can be. No, they probably won't guess DI per se, they won't ask if they came from a sperm bank. But they can pick up tensions, silences, whispered asides, funny looks. A first child will also notice more concrete things if DI is again part of your life, as he observes your efforts to have a second child.

There are a number of books for parents and children that can help at this stage. If you are disclosing DI, *Flight of the Stork* clarifies for parents how children process information about reproduction.[15] *How I Began* was the first DI-specific children's book, written in 1988 by Australian social workers.[16] In 1991 two British DI moms wrote *My Story*, which begins with Mummy and Daddy's sadness, then tells of their happiness after a pregnancy happens with help from a doctor and some very kind men who give their sperm.[17] In *Mommy, Did I Grow in Your Tummy?*, a married couple go to the doctor for help, and in vitro fertilization (IVF), donor egg, donor sperm, surrogacy, and adoption are outlined.[18] Similarly, *Where Did I Really Come From?* looks at all the ways to add babies to families.[19] If you used these children's books earlier, to prepare yourself or to talk with your preschooler, you may find your school-age child now interested in reading them on her own.

Whether or not you're now talking about DI, you can lay the groundwork that will help your child become more prepared to accept family differences. Some books focus on family diversity.[20] If your child notices differences, books can help you talk about them positively.[21] In *Play Ball, Zachary*, a boy is good at reading and painting, but his dad wants him to play sports, and they work this out.[22] Books on self-esteem build the confidence children need to feel lovable just as they are.[23] You may want to seek out books celebrating father-child bonds.[24] Moms may feel a bit left out if this goes overboard, but dads deserve some special attention.

When Your Child Is a Preteen

The preteen phase is your opportunity for telling or for more in-depth discussions before adolescent issues hit. For children who already know of DI and for children who are just learning of their origins, this is a time when a deeper understanding is possible. At this age a child can come to understand what genetic relatedness does and doesn't mean, and how her family feels about it. He can realize it was sad and painful for his dad not to have sperm, even though he was much happier once he got such a great kid. A preteen child may have interesting questions about who the donor was and what his motivations were. But DI may also be treated quite casually sometimes. Peggy Orenstein interviewed one very open family for her article in the *New York Times Magazine*.

> Gabe, one of three brothers conceived through DI, explains what he knows about the circumstances of his birth. "We're from a sperm bank," the 10-year-old says, matter-of-factly. Before turning back to the TV, he adds that he'd like to meet the man someday: "It would be cool."[25]

It may take a while for DI to sink in, for a preteen to connect up pieces of conversations, bits of information, and form a more complete picture of DI. Rebecca and Lawrence had agreed they'd both look for opportunities to talk with Ashley. Topics would come close, but she'd shift to something else, like the part of the story where she was born, not the beginning where she was conceived. Rebecca was alone with Ashley when their talk got more in-depth. Rebecca explains:

This occurred when Ashley was around eight years old, in third grade. We were sitting on the sofa, and Ashley was expressing a sense of disappointment that her cat wasn't having kittens. At that point I said, "Gee, Ashley, maybe Peaches is infertile." Ashley asked what that meant, and I said, "Like Daddy and me." I thought this was the golden opportunity, the opening we had been looking for to bring up with Ashley the issue of donor insemination. "You know Daddy and I have infertility problems," which she did know since that was part of our decision to adopt Jordan, our son.

I went on to explain that in our situation, it's like gardening, there are seeds you put in the ground to grow. When you have children, the men have sperm that grow in the mother's womb. Daddy's seeds didn't grow; there was something wrong with his sperm. Ashley asked what was wrong with the seeds. I said they didn't work right, so we went to the doctor and he found somebody with good seeds and put those inside Mommy. "And it worked! And, that's how we had you." Her first response was something we didn't expect—"Did that make Daddy sad?"

The topic of DI didn't resurface often. Rebecca remembers:

One day she came home from health class after the sex education talk and asked me, "Do you and Daddy use condoms?" Once again I gathered my thoughts and started, "Honey, remember Daddy doesn't have any sperm?" and this time it brought out more questions. "Then how did you have me?" I explained, and it helped that we'd been active in RESOLVE. She knew kids, in addition to Jordan, who had been adopted, so she understood their dads are their dads even though they have another biological parent. She asked if she could meet the donor and I told her we didn't know who he was but our doctor knew him. I told her her dad would be glad to talk more about DI, but we wanted to leave that up to her.

For the next two weeks she spent extra time telling her dad how much she loved him. She didn't really bring it up till a year later, when she made a joke about not having to worry about having his allergies. And then the next day she went and asked him if he was OK with her making a joke about that. She's a great kid and seems OK with it, but she hasn't yet told any of her friends. So we're glad we were very reserved all these years, only sharing it with our parents' group.

If you're telling your child for the first time at this stage, it may be because you know he'll understand the concept of privacy. Modesty about one's body, discretion, self-protection, and loyalty in keeping a secret for a close friend are all issues that a preteen is trying to learn to manage. The ability to understand privacy allows you to tell your child of DI, to tell him whom you've confided in, to give him your assurance that he, too, can confide in anyone he's close to. He might need help to understand that certain family members or friends aren't aware because you were concerned that they might have beliefs that would make them scared or disapproving of DI. Although it might be painful for you to have withheld this from family members you couldn't trust, he may be quite glad if such people don't know about his DI conception; he can then have some control over how to proceed. This age group tends to know a lot about discrimination, prejudice, ignorance, and meanness from the playground to the evening news.[26] They can understand, with some help from parents, that you can feel great about something but choose not to share it with others who have been insensitive about other issues.

This is an important stage to draw out some of the more complex issues. At age five, you could leave the story at "seeds" or a "nice man helped." But now you want your child to understand a few more concepts before going into the fray of adolescence. You want her to know that DI is a very common family-building choice, kept quiet partly because it's just so easy to keep private, but probably about as common as adoption. Because these years can be a time of discomfort with topics the child perceives to be sexual or embarrassing, she may have a negative reaction to sperm banks, masturbation, or semen analysis. "That's disgusting!" is a normal reaction for this age group. It's important to convey a positive image of sperm donors, that they're carefully selected and as a group are smart, open-minded, healthy, and good young men.

Many parents nowadays have more information about their specific donor and need to decide in what way to make this available to their children. You may already have an opinion about the ideal time to show your child the information you got from the sperm bank. If your plan was to wait until much later, after your child is comfortable with her self-image, but she wants to learn all the details now, you may want to ask her for some time to think over how best to share so much information—then check on those counseling resources.

It's just as likely, however, that your child will ask for less information than you anticipated. You want her to understand that you're glad to talk further, that ongoing discussions are expected and a good sign, and that she can talk to others if she'd like to. If you've already met other DI parents, you can offer to plan a get-together so that she can be around other kids who know about DI too. She may want to correspond or e-mail with other kids conceived via DI. You can tell her it's fine to be curious about donors too. She might want to write to the sperm bank to let them know she's curious about her donor; if her donor is known, she might want to ask him how he's felt about donating the sperm that led to her birth. But it's more likely that a preteen will quietly ponder all this without taking any action. If she has your blessing to someday learn more if and when she needs to, she can then choose whether or not to bring it up with you. If she goes off and privately learns about DI as a teenager, she may be less worried about hurting you or violating family rules if you've told her you want her to do whatever she needs to do to feel at peace with her origins.

One family tells the kind of story that parents worry will be awful, but this family handled it well. DI is a frequent topic in their household, since both parents offer DI phone support through RESOLVE. At age ten, Kate was mad at her father for having to give their dog away. Her visiting cousin asked how she could be so mean to her father. Kate replied, "Oh, no, he's not part of me. I came from a donor, I don't have any of him in me. He's my evil stepfather." Kate's father, Troy, was taken aback and unsure what to say, especially in front of this cousin. He said, "You're being rough. Does your cousin know what you're talking about?" She said, "Yes, we saw *The Fresh Prince of Bel Aire.*" Troy later learned there was an episode about DI, but this cousin didn't know Kate was a DI child. They discussed it so that everyone would understand. Troy realized his daughter was just trying to push his buttons, to test him, but it really shocked him. "She rocked me back. I wasn't expecting to deal with comments like this just yet, not when she's only ten. I thought it would happen when she was a teenager." He later took her aside and let her know she had hurt his feelings, not by what she'd said but the way she'd said it. "You don't have to be so rough with me. My feelings can get hurt just like yours."

Most family discussions won't be so dramatic! There are some topics that you and your child can read about and talk over. *Let Me Explain* is ideal for this age group; a girl and her dad are two of a kind except for her genes, which came from a donor.[27] *How Babies and Families Are Made*, emphasizing positive differences in families, reviews reproduction and anatomy. DI is presented as the first family-building alternative to intercourse, even before IVF.[28]

This is a good time to call upon your inner circle of loved ones who know your child well and have been willing to learn about DI, or a professional specialized in DI counseling and able to get to know your child. Especially as your child moves toward adolescence, she needs other adults she can trust, as she may need to declare her independence from you or be more comfortable discussing this topic with others.

When Your Child Is an Adolescent

Adolescence is difficult for most parents, for reasons that have nothing to do with DI. Most adolescents are preoccupied with their own identity, appearance, feelings, desires, peers, and so on. Adolescence is a time when children recognize parents' weak spots and may use this knowledge hurtfully as they work out their own issues. You may worry your adolescent could use his knowledge of DI origins against you. But it's just as likely that your fear of this will lead you to overcompensate in some way. You may be overly permissive, trying too hard to be and do what your teen wants in order to avoid that rejection. Instead, you need to be prepared to be the confident one, the voice of reason and truth, even if you can't always keep that voice calm. Troy writes:

> Will they one day, in the great teenage battles of the future, hurl some obscene statement at me in anger, such as "Hey, Dad, get f——ed, you're not my father anyway." I'm sure of it. Will I wilt up in my corner and be blown away? No way. They know who their dad is. They'll just want to say it to see what happens.

You can't let dreaded statements like "I wish you'd never had me" be crushing. If that type of statement is ever said, you can discuss it later, but for right then, "I'm your parent, for better or worse" and "The rule still is x" or "We agreed to y" or "It's time to do z." Karen has played this out many times in her mind.

> We treat the kids no differently than we would if we hadn't had any problems. . . . We anticipate that one day one of the kids may get mad at Joseph and say, "You're not my father!" when he grounds them or takes the keys to the car away. If that day comes, we'll deal with it just as we've dealt with everything else in life. At this point we anticipate that anything can happen when raising a teenager.

But do kids make hurtful allusions to DI? Do they play this card that everyone fears could be so damaging? Teens usually hurt you because their verbal skills have caught up with their ability to perceive parental vulnerabilities, but their ability to control their feelings and words isn't so well developed. Nevertheless, they aren't usually cruel, vicious, calculating monsters. They're more likely to focus on the everyday devastation of your self-esteem, like commenting on your hairstyle, something more immediately important to them as they struggle with their own issues, such as their attractiveness.

When you worry about what might be said to you, you're forgetting that teens are more focused on themselves than on their parents. Many have confused feelings about some aspect of their identity. Teens search for clues to figure out who they are, why they're valuable, who they'll become, who they're like, who they're close to. Given DI, they often have a very big piece of missing or limited information. It's not impossible that they'll find this intriguing, sort of like having purple hair. But it's very possible they'll find it a confusing factor in any areas of uncertainty they have about themselves. Or they could use the donor as a positive source of fantasy, building him up to be handsome, brilliant, athletic, and so on. You may watch as some of your hardest work in building your child's skills and self-confidence gets attributed to the donor during a stage of adolescence.

Dads can understandably feel threatened by a child's positive view of the donor. No matter what your child does or doesn't express, you may feel a resurgence of envy of the donor, envy that was first triggered by the donor's fertility. You may worry that you're not as brilliant as the donor and attribute your child's academic success to the donor's SAT scores, not your years of help with study habits and school projects. You probably once felt a lot handsomer than you do now, but you need to realize the donor may have lost his hair and his waistline too!

You need to be sure you aren't projecting your own issues and worries onto your adolescent. You may presume he thinks the donor is a cooler guy than you when he's not thinking about the donor much at all. But he may well think of himself as the smart one, without crediting all your hours of homework help *or* the donor's genes! As parents sum up the teenage years, "Who needs an encyclopedia—I have a thirteen-year-old!" It's a natural time for a child to be full of himself and not at all aware of how amazing his parents are. If your son is putting you down and himself up, don't assume it has anything to do with all those superlative things you chose in a donor and responsibly told him about a couple of years ago. He may just be being a teenager, bragging to fill out a vulnerable ego, unaware that parents aren't always so immune to identity crises either.

Adolescence can also be worrisome for you if some of the information you have about the donor isn't positive. You may be very uncertain about when to disclose all you know, now or in adulthood, when your child may have a better perspective on the context and interpretation of the information you're worried about. The most common example is related to flippant answers by donors on long profiles, also discussed in chapter 3. If a donor casually wrote that he became a donor "for the cash," he wasn't thinking how that might sound to a teenager. If you were able to get thorough, nonidentifying information before choosing a donor, you may have felt quite pleased with your choice until you realized your intellectual daughter thinks athletes are blockheads and athletics was the donor's major source of identity—at least during the year he filled out his donor profile. From the serious to the very trivial, you may worry, and you need to have a safe place to express those worries. Once again, the goal is to free yourself of your anxieties so that you can concentrate on responding in a supportive way to the very unpredictable reaction your child will have to a deeper level of information about the donor.

Perhaps you have not talked with your child about the donor because you fear you have so little to tell. For parents of children born in the 1980s, it was unusual to get extensive nonidentifying information, and parents-to-be weren't fully informed of available options. If you acknowledge your child's pain, if you take responsibility for any options you ignored or rights you were unable to protect, your child can grieve the losses and accept the painful lack of genetic information.

Becky decided to be very proactive on behalf of her children, seeking out more information on their two donors. She feared that if she waited until they were young adults able to take on the task themselves, the donor might be less motivated or even unable to be located. She shares the story of the steps she took:

I have a son, Brandon, who will be 15 this year. He was conceived via the Xytex bank in Georgia. I have twins, Lindsey and Jeremy, who will soon be 13, conceived via Idant in New York. Two or three years ago I began to try to see if I could get some more background information on the donors for my kids. I have no desire to upset the donor's wish for anonymity. I just ask that he try to realize that a child needs to know more about their biological dad than just his hair color, eye color, height, weight, blood type, and nationality. This is all I had on Brandon's donor. On the twins, I did have a list of his hobbies and field of study. My children have all shown that they need to know about the people in their "family" as a part of knowing who they are. They have all relished stories of ancestors they have never met because they died long ago, but who have shown up in school reports over the years. To know yourself, you need to know where you came from. It gives you roots.

With some personnel changes, my requests via the phone to Xytex fell into a hole twice. Last fall, however, Xytex considered my request and sent a letter to the last-known address of the donor, asking him to complete the questions they now ask donors and the questions I specifically asked. My questions were based on observations of my son and questions a counselor told me would eventually come up. The letter was returned, as the donor no longer lived there. I was then asked if I would pay a nominal amount for Xytex to make a more extensive search. I agreed. Within just a few days, the donor was found. Xytex talked to him over the phone. He had recently gotten married and his spouse was out of town. My letter and Xytex's questionnaire were sent to him. With his spouse gone, he said he would sit down that weekend and reply. I also sent a picture of Brandon for his comments.

I told Brandon the letter was coming and warned him that most donors answer that they became a donor "for the money," so he wouldn't feel upset. The letter came one evening when I was en route to take my daughter to gymnastics. I gave it to Brandon and told him we could discuss it when I returned. Brandon kind of "grunted" as he continued with his reading. When I got back, the letter was laid by my purse. He immediately came out of his bedroom and acted relieved. He now knows why he has a "substantial" nose and sees his height is in line with his donor dad. He was disappointed that his donor wasn't a baseball fan. However, he thought he might check out tennis and golf to see if he would like them like his donor. The donor did a wonderful job of answering the questions and telling Brandon how lucky he is. He commented that Brandon didn't look like him, but that he was a fine-looking young man. This is all that Brandon needed. He doesn't show any signs of wanting to meet his donor. That could change one day. I have left information with Xytex on how they can contact me, should the donor become interested in meeting.

When I initially called Idant, they indicated that they would not try to reach the donor. We could put a letter in his file, if we would like, in case the donor became interested some day. My daughter, in particular, is upset that Brandon got information and she can't get any. Her donor is Jewish. This weekend, Lindsey went to a Jewish ceremony with excitement so she could learn about her donor's faith. I have just gotten from Idant a brochure of the information they provide on donors now. I plan to ask for all such information on the twins' donor. Then, I plan to approach them to do for the twins what Xytex did for Brandon.

My kids are comfortable with how they were born, and I have an open communication with them. There isn't anything they won't ask me. They know I tell the truth. It the midst of hormones and teenage years, I must have that to help my kids cope. I don't believe in relationships built on lies. Secrets don't work well in families. They are always found out, at the wrong time, and with the wrong person telling them.

DI can be a very difficult issue if your teen is finding out about it for the first time now, when her development is challenging enough.[29] This is especially true if she senses that you're telling her for your needs, not for hers. Most distressing is if you didn't tell her yourself but someone else slipped. Many of the upset adults speaking out against DI were told quite dysfunctionally. Take care in choosing the right time and the right reason for telling. If you've waited this long, you may as well wait until you're telling for your child's needs, not your own. Margaret's mother felt she had to disclose her DI conception when Margaret was sixteen because Margaret was trying to reestablish contact with her father after years of estrangement. Margaret was upset that many others had been told before her. She remembers:

> Even though I was bitter that everyone but me seemed to know, I could understand my parents' compulsion to tell other adults in the family about my conception so as to waylay any suspicions of adultery since my father had had a vasectomy some years before. I didn't get to express my fury that cousins only five years older than me knew about this. It seemed the information was passed down through the family as though everyone had some right or reason to know about it. The utter disregard for my feelings and my privacy left me feeling a sense of betrayal far deeper than that one page [her *Newsweek* essay] could allow me to express. I also didn't have room to say that even though I am not biologically linked to my father's family, I love them all dearly and couldn't imagine life without them.

If you aren't planning on telling your child of DI until adulthood, you may become uncomfortable or downright anxious every time a discussion topic comes close to genetics, fertility, sperm, or the like. You may also be uncomfortable whenever your family comes close to anyone who "knows," which is especially difficult if many loved ones do know. Everyone in your inner circle of confidants may begin to feel bad as other adult topics begin to be shared with this young person. You'll need to be prepared to someday explain why you didn't tell during adolescence. It will help if you can re-create your decision-making process, to describe why you envisioned adulthood as the better time for disclosure. For now, you need to make sure any feelings of paranoia that your child will "find out" don't cast a shadow over your relationship with your child.

When Your Child Becomes an Adult

By the time you're trying to shift from a parental role to an adult-to-adult relationship with your child, DI may be a topic first discussed years ago, or it may be a topic you're trying to find the "right" time to raise, or it may be a topic you never intend to discuss with your child. Obviously these raise very different issues, but you will benefit from this section no matter what your circumstances.

It's possible that some of the parents choosing to read this book will be intending never to tell their child, and these parents need support. But trying to hide our bias as authors toward telling, preferably before adolescence, would be foolish. We know there are many parents who feel that this information can only be damaging, yet there still may come a time when you decide to share it with your child. One woman tells the story of nursing her own mother through a terminal illness and feeling so close, able to share anything—and wanting her child to have that same sense of total connection. This was her turning point in deciding not to take the DI secret to her grave, and once she decided that, she could focus on when and how to tell.

If you plan to keep donor insemination confidential, you may benefit from discussing again as a couple how this decision, made years ago, fits in with your new stage of family life. You need to sort out when and how your choice to be private even from an adult child does, or doesn't, strain you personally, maritally, or in your efforts to develop a friendship with your adult child, as well as when it does, or doesn't, feel like a relief and an appropriate protection of your child. For all parents it's vital to be honest with yourself and with your inner circle, because if you aren't fine with DI or able to comfortably admit in what way you are not fine, your child will sense that and may misinterpret it.

Our goal, both in writing this book and in our counseling, is to change social attitudes toward DI so much that if you do tell, you can feel more confident that your child will ultimately view this news positively, not negatively. It may never be OK that there was so little

donor information provided or that your family began with such suffering for the parents, but you'll certainly get across just how wanted
your child was. And it can be liberating to have communication and
trust between family members. Although you may fear that telling
carries too great a risk of harm, lifelong withholding of this information from your child, who has become your friend, must be seen as a
significant burden for you, and for your relationship, to bear.

If you told your child years ago and the topic submerged or has been
very seldom mentioned, it may help to consider what new adult-level
topics you could raise, deepening your family's understanding of DI.
Trying to initiate talks about DI may not be easy. This can have very
little to do with DI or your family's loving connection per se. Young
adults are still working hard to get distance from you, to leave family
issues and dependency behind. Old communication patterns may color
how you feel about discussing any topic of such complexity and inti-
macy. You could fear you're pushing or intruding on your child if you
raise the topic—and vice versa. It doesn't really matter how those
dynamics got started in the past by you or by your child; you just may
not be willing to risk a bad scene over such a pivotal issue in your
relationship. It might help to set aside an agreed-upon time, maybe with
the help of someone who can ease any tension, pain, or awkwardness.
Maybe it will help to imagine regular, briefer talks, to practice slowly
wading into comfort with the topic.

If you're just now telling your child, you'll want to talk to those
DI families who have had ongoing conversations as a family, because
they can help you anticipate what issues you may need to bring up and
what complex questions your child might ask you to address. You'll
certainly need time to talk with your child, time chosen when you
think he might best be able to process the information. If you're telling your child because you feel the pressure of some upcoming event,
such as his move far away for a couple of years, try to organize yourself to tell him long before this event so he won't forever link the
memory of DI's disclosure to a time of stressful change.

Certainly try to tell your child in a way that isn't confused with issues already loaded for her. If, for example, you and your spouse are separating and she's already angry with you about that, this wouldn't be an ideal time to tell! She might feel constrained from expressing her feelings, knowing the stress you are already experiencing, or conversely, she might lash out with accumulated anger, seemingly about DI but actually regarding the overall stress the family is in. It would also be unfair to risk marring or stressing a time that's meant to be very happy and fun, such as the birth of your grandchild. It might seem like a good time to explain genetics or how you felt about appearance comments when she was born—that will certainly be on your mind. But your child deserves to have her needs be the focus, if at all possible, and for you to pick a more neutral, calm time in her life to disclose DI.

Most parents who wait until their child's adulthood to disclose DI are terrified of his anger. Your child may very well be angry or hurt at not having been told sooner. Any emotional reaction requires your acknowledgment, not defense of your behavior and decisions. Later you can explain, share the journal described earlier in this chapter, or offer the input of your inner circle who have known how hard you've struggled with whether and when to tell. Gary offers this example from a journal he and his wife are keeping for their child:

> Right now at this very moment, I am scared to death that you love me less because of what you've read in this book. I feel like crying. How do I explain? How do I make you understand I AM your dad! I love you so much. At this stage in our lives, without the donor you wouldn't be here reading this.

During the initial discussions, you need to give your child the message that you can handle her reaction, whatever it is. If your child knows you love her and recognizes that this was hard for you too, the anger will lessen over time. Losses acknowledged and shared help relationships grow. Your child will need you to accept all her negative feelings and not force her to express positive feelings if premature or not genuine.

But she'll eventually need to know that you did believe in DI, look positively on how you conceived her, and love her for who she is. You also may need to have information on hand for her. If she has really been sheltered from the infertility world totally, she may know as little about DI as you did when you first heard about it.

The stage of telling again involves the risk of wider openness about DI than you might have preferred. Your willingness to lose control over who knows is an important message to a young adult. If he wants to tell his story to Oprah, ideally you prepare to meet Oprah, or at least wish him well in doing so if you agree it's not for you. This information now becomes your child's. He needs to respect how you've dealt with it, even if he would have handled it radically differently. His initial opinions may change as he lives with the information for a while too.

THOSE CONCEIVED VIA DI SHARE THEIR VIEWS

We don't yet have lots of stories from adults told of their DI origins. Those at peace with DI are often too busy with other life challenges to stop and make DI a priority. Much of what you may have heard about children's responses are stories of pain and anger.[30] Unfortunately, this is what sells magazines and TV advertising. One article that got tremendous attention appeared in the *New York Times Magazine*.[31] Tom Riordan, reviewing the article for RESOLVE of NYC, questioned its value for others conceived with the help of DI.

> Orenstein uses the stories of a Utah man and California woman to illustrate how grown children with brutal and uncaring parents may use fantasy to distance themselves. These two people, fleeing bad parents, call the sperm donors whose sperm their parents used to conceive them "father."
>
> But Orenstein does children conceived with donor sperm a grave disservice. No one blames marital intercourse when parents beat or neglect children so conceived, yet Orenstein blames her two interviewees' suffering on donor insemination (DI) and the secrecy often surrounding

it. . . . DI itself is no more a problem than being Iranian or Jewish or having a small penis or the wrong size breasts. The problem is other people's attitude about such features. Our sperm donor is an important figure in our family, and he may well become a significant person in our family after identifying information becomes available to our son at age 18. But this man is not our son's father, and Ms. Orenstein should not generalize the point of view of two people traumatized by their parents when she is describing so many other normal parents and children. It is bad journalism and leaves a misanthropic taste in the mouth. If DI feels threatening to her in some way, Orenstein would do better to write a personal essay exploring her situation, and not pretend knowledge of my heart or my son's. Her attitude does threaten us.[32]

It may be that those conceived via DI need to begin telling their own stories, free of the complications of producers, reporters, talk show hosts, and editors who have varying degrees of knowledge about donor insemination, as well as their own agendas. Sometimes the portrait the reader or viewer ends up with may not be exactly what the DI adults wished to convey. In the worst cases they're made to look obsessive about their genetic background and insensitive to their parents. One reporter describes Donor Offspring, a small organization founded by a Missouri woman.

Donor Offspring . . . claims that since 1981 it has attracted tormented souls. . . . Candace Turner . . . works the Donahue–Hard Copy circuit and tends toward theatrical hyperbole ("All donor-insemination babies have been emotionally, sexually or physically abused").[33]

Bill Cordray, who was focused on in Orenstein's article and was once active in Donor Offspring, feels the media have often overemphasized the negatives about his family life, making him sound angrier and unhappier than he is about DI. He has worked hard for reform, often through adoptee rights organizations, not only in his home state but also by speaking worldwide. He hopes someday soon there'll be a forum, such as an e-mail list, to help people worldwide with different perspectives on DI learn from each other.[34]

Ironically, adults speaking out against traumatic family secrets scare many parents into concealing DI because it seems to have been so distressing. We want to also share positive stories, those the media find boring, because they may encourage parents that DI can be shared as a family. There are many adults coping well with DI origins, but they're still unlikely to go public. Children close to their dads have felt the stigma and ignorance have been too great to share their story. (This might explain why so many of the adults speaking out have a dad who is estranged from them.) We hope more families will speak out together, with less fear of negative ramifications.

Sue tells how she found out about DI after coming home from college. She noticed her mother was acting "pretty weird," as if something was bothering her.

> After fumbling for the right words, she told me that the man who I thought was my father was not my biological father. Before she could explain herself, my mind started to race. Who was my father? The milkman? The mailman? The METER READER? She started crying and somehow was able to explain that my father was sterile and they could never have had children in the conventional way. Without getting into much detail about the whole procedure, my mother explained that she had heard of a clinic that did artificial insemination.
>
> Now, being that this happened twenty-some-odd years ago when the whole idea of artificial insemination was fairly new and unheard of, my mother decided to tell no one about the procedure. Because being artificially inseminated required a trip to a faraway clinic, my mother fibbed to everyone and told them she was going to some hospital to have her gallbladder removed and it just so happened she got pregnant in that same period of time.
>
> To say that I was completely stunned is to put it lightly. It's really strange to discover that the person who you've always thought was one of your parents really isn't. But it was actually very relieving in many

ways. I have an older brother who is adopted and I'd never understood why my parents had adopted if they could have their own children. I had always wondered where I got my unique eye and hair color that no one else on the other side of my family had.

My mother left it to me to tell whomever I wanted. I don't feel that it's such a secret. I have found, however, that telling people how I was conceived usually makes other people uncomfortable, but most are accepting of it.

One regret Sue still has is that she would have liked more medical information and to know the nationality of the donor. She jokes, saying she's "half Italian and half Pyrex." But she has positive feelings about DI as well.

First of all, being a DI child has really made me feel like a wanted child. I was not a mistake. Second, I'm also really aware of the fertility problems that others face. Now that I am an adult, I am involved in an egg donor program, kind of as my own way to help out those who want to have a child just as badly as my mother did so many years ago. . . . I can tell you that only positive results will occur. There's no feeling as wonderful as knowing your parents love you so much before you were even conceived that they'd do anything they could to bring you into this world.

Karen writes:

My parents are great. They didn't make a big deal about how or when to tell me about my origins—there was no big session where they sat me down and told me I was different. Instead, their method seemed to be simply to wait until I asked questions and then tell me the whole truth. What could be more natural? Luckily for them, I was an inquisitive kid, but I believe it was my parents' forthright but casual attitude that made this completely a nonissue for me. . . .

I remember thinking that I would just like to see a picture of the donor, to see if I looked like him (my scientific curiosity already in place), but I certainly didn't obsess about finding him. I also remember thinking that it was pretty cool that I wasn't conceived like everybody else. Unlike the outward show of uniformity and normality necessary in a school playground (like the right brand of jeans), I knew this was something different and even special about me that I could keep inside and share or hide as I wished. Instinctively, I guess I didn't talk much about it, since it fell under the same taboo category as thinking about your parents having sex. . . . Maybe I would be more interested in him if there were any way to find him, but I gather at that time no records were kept at all. . . .

I don't feel any psychological "loss" for not knowing the source of half of my chromosomes. . . . I know my parents wanted me very much. As an older teenager, I don't recall ever thinking about the donor or my father's infertility. My life was pretty busy and exciting in late high school and into university. So when my parents phoned me in my third year at Queen's to ask if I were willing to speak to an Ottawa infertility support group with them, I was surprised—mostly because I hadn't thought about it in so long, but also because I didn't know what on earth I would have to say, other than "No, this hasn't affected me."[35]

She later writes:

DI is such a "nonissue" for me that it feels strange to get this much attention for it! It is not at all a part of any definition of my "self." Anyway, I'm glad to answer questions, but I don't feel any need to be in contact with other DI offspring.

One fourteen-year-old, interviewed by a reporter, also emphasized that DI is a nonissue:

It's not a big deal. . . . I do what all kids do. I go to school. . . . I have friends. I'm going to have a bat mitzvah. How I got here doesn't change anything. This is the way I was born, and that's it.[36]

But there certainly can be challenges for those conceived via DI. Monica only learned of DI in her thirties; her family isn't open to ongoing discussions. She writes:

I always thought I was adopted, mostly because my dad and I look so different. But then my mom had the bracelet from the hospital, so I had to believe I wasn't adopted. There were subtle clues—like there was no talk of his side of the family. I do respect my mom; DI was so groundbreaking back then, she had so much audacity to have a pregnancy this way, and she wanted kids so much. My mom says my dad was supportive when they were deciding, said he'd love the baby. Many men need guidance in parenting but my mom deferred to my dad because she felt bad about his infertility and about DI. It's hard to know what role DI played in our family's problems; I don't think DI was his only problem! But I wish I'd known sooner. . . .

My parents divorced when I was eight. I have a younger brother, conceived with a different donor. Mom told each of us by phone, not that long ago. She was afraid we were about to hear it elsewhere.

Mom never was good at talking about feelings; she was in denial about my wanting more information about the donor. She told me, "Make up your father, he's whoever you imagine him to be." I think ultimately her telling us will bring us closer together.

Margaret Brown found out about her DI conception at sixteen, nine years after her parents' divorce. In a 1995 *Newsweek* article she describes the dramatic lack of information from the fresh sperm days.

I'm a person created by donor insemination, someone who will never know half of her identity. I feel anger and confusion and I'm filled with questions. Whose eyes do I have? Why the big secret? Who gave my family the idea that my biological roots are not important? To deny someone the knowledge of his or her biological origins is dreadfully wrong. . . . Parents must realize that all the love and attention in the world can't mask that underlying, almost subconscious feeling that something is askew. I greatly appreciate the sacrifices my mother has made and the love my family has given me. But even while being enveloped in my father's sister's warmest embrace, I feel a strange little twinge of something deep inside me—like I'm borrowing someone else's family.[37]

She faced added feelings stirred by the many people who contacted her after her article appeared, and sent us a follow-up.

> Both my mom and I are sick with all the hype resulting from the *Newsweek* piece. . . . It was really frustrating having people interview me expecting some sort of major controversy. They weren't interested in me or the fact that I'm a normal person; they're interested in this weird way of making babies and they expect me to be a freak with five arms and two heads or something. . . .
>
> I don't want to camp out on anyone's doorstep, or even have a relationship with my donor, for that matter. I already have a family; I don't need another one. I am an adult, I'm in school, and I'm quite happy with my life as it is. I would just like to satisfy my curiosity about the man who passed his genes on to me. I just want to ask a few questions—no, not even that—maybe just be a bystander, a fly on the wall, in his life for a day. Maybe I could search pictures of his family to see if I resemble any of them. . . . I asked a good friend if she thought I should have been told. She replied matter-of-factly, "You needed to know, your soul needed the truth."

It can be annoying or amusing at times to be at the center of controversy, with parents and professionals concerned over your every distress. Margaret reflects on the terminology of DI.

> "DI offspring" brings visions of seal babies on the Discovery Channel. . . . "Those conceived by DI" is a mouthful. . . . Basically, the "DI child" is just like any other kid . . . they watch cartoons, they cry when it thunders loud, they don't like to eat their vegetables.

Adults conceived via DI face significant losses with donor anonymity, which may be greatly eased for children now. Greater societal acceptance would also go a long way toward easing DI's challenges.

Parenting with Resolution

Your own feelings and ideas about DI will change drastically over time. You'll continue to have new challenges and insights as both you and your children grow—unless you block that process, forcing your opinions and reactions to lock into one position, one approach, one ideology. The bottom line on helping your children deal with DI is being at ease and confident with the issues yourself. If you've found peace with your choices in conceiving your children, they're more likely to follow your lead.

Family members may not frequently think of DI, but when you do, you'll know you can continue a dialog begun with love, commitment, and courage. Troy explains:

> It takes time to feel totally comfortable with the whole DI process. If I had it to do it over again, I'd choose those sperm banks that allow the child to contact the donor when they turn eighteen. The longer I spend with my children, the less my being biologically connected to them is a concern for me. I am their father, father figure, dad, committed caregiver, all of the above. I don't have to be convinced of any of that anymore. I'm too busy being IT. My concern is only for my kids, to give them the help and support they need, in ALL areas. . . . And in the long and short of it, any biological connections we don't have is a sadness we share. But then again, what the hell is so damn special about my genes that I can't make up for in doing the best I can in the nurturing department? Simply put, it's not the part of myself I give a lot of thought or credit to.
>
> My eagerness and possible talents in nurturing my two children to the utmost is the part of me that I hope they will take with them through their lives and perhaps find useful in the creation of their own families. Being the gleeful instigator in the dispersion of sperm is easy, for those that can or have it. Being a father is the hard part. If someone told me they could fix me so as to have my "own biological kids" tomorrow, I wouldn't even be interested. I have two of my own now.

Chapter Eight

Changing Families,
Different Challenges

When we decided to make Helping the Stork *a book for everyone turning to DI, not just infertile couples, we took some heat over including unmarried moms. Some said our book would never sell in conservative areas of America. Well, anyone turning to DI has already had to question the traditional meaning of "family."*

I think young people now know families come in many shapes and sizes. My friend who lives in a small town far from my own liberal Massachusetts told me of a conversation over dinner with her preteen children. One piped up, "You know, I heard two teachers had a baby together—two women teachers! They did it that way . . . I forget what it's called. Oh yeah, internal rejuvenation."

She was not only pretty close, but she added a positive twist!

—Carol

While most writing on DI, the prior chapters in this book included, focuses on first-time married couples who turn to donor insemination to have children, there are others considering and using DI to build their families as well. It's important to acknowledge that some DI experiences are different when your family structure doesn't quite resemble Beaver Cleaver's family. Fortunately, the 1950s' view of family is passing. Families are formed in many

195

ways, and families of many different varieties are finding acceptance in a society that is certainly growing more tolerant of, if not always embracing, diversity. Much has been written on single moms, lesbian moms, stepfamilies, and families after divorce, so our goal here is to highlight how donor insemination might play out somewhat differently for these families.

You might choose to read just the section of this chapter that applies to you. But if you'll look at the other sections, we think you'll find there's much to be learned by looking at DI from different perspectives as well.

BECOMING A MOM WITHOUT A DAD

Single women and lesbian couples face some common challenges as they move toward parenthood with DI. While a married couple has the luxury (or the burden, some might say) of choosing to limit any awareness of their unusual conception approach to an inner circle of confidants, unmarried women find most everyone will be curious about how their pregnancy got started. Parents-to-be differ in how comfortable they are with revealing or concealing information about what they've been through. But no matter where you fall on the openness/privacy continuum, you may find yourself at a loss for smooth, easy words to suit every occasion you'll encounter once pregnant and parenting.

At some point you're bound to face the judgment of those who think children should always be raised by heterosexual couples. Even if harsh judgments come from only a small percentage of loved ones or acquaintances, with many others approving or at least accepting of your choice, it's a worry for women, who often can't tell who will hold which attitudes.

Although you may be prepared to deal with unsupportive acquaintances, you might be surprised to find you have to deal with judgmental medical professionals as well. Until recent years, even in major cities, unmarried women were routinely refused access to DI services. This has begun to change because of fears of discrimination charges, if not belief in women's reproductive rights. But it still may take some effort to locate a supportive medical team. As one medical review puts it:

> Physicians in the U.S. have often withheld artificial donor insemination from unmarried women because of fears of psychological damage to the children. . . . Doctors are also concerned that the women are emotionally abnormal, selfish, or have "something against men." Lesbians have been especially suspect.[1]

Some doctors will evaluate you to be "sure" your child won't be at financial or emotional risk, even if they don't request such reassurance from married patients.

You might think the obvious "solution" is to turn to home insemination with a known donor, and many have. But in addition to the medical concerns with fresh sperm raised throughout this book, unmarried women take on added legal risks. As Laura Benkov, author of *Reinventing the Family*, notes:

> Significantly, in many states, the donors' lack of parental status hinges on medical mediation. That is, donors who directly give sperm to women can be, and often are, legally considered parents. . . . People creating families through donor insemination do so most safely—that is, with least threat to their integrity as a family unit—if they utilize medical help.[2]

No matter what your original intentions, a known donor may be viewed as a dad if he wants to expand his role or when some legal authority expands his responsibilities because you're unable to care for all your child's needs. Even if you work with a lawyer to draft a statement of your intentions as you begin inseminations, you have no legal guarantees.[3]

It may be a disturbing compromise to work with a medical team and an anonymous donor in order to protect yourself from bad outcomes, especially if you've wanted pregnancy to begin more naturally or positively. But supportive medical teams can be found through women's health care centers or through the organizations listed in the Resources section of this book. Also, you may decide to educate the local doctor, helping future DI moms-to-be. You can work with a progressive bank offering you more peace of mind as you select a donor. Your Trying Times may more quickly end in pregnancy with a medical team guiding you through inseminations.

A difficult stage for DI moms is when their child first notices not having a daddy or first feels bad about the difference. You might find it tempting to slip into a family view of the donor as a dad. It can be painful to acknowledge that your child, who does have a genetic heritage he can be proud of, nevertheless faces the loss of a daddy. Coping with your own feelings and then focusing on what your child might need to heal is brilliantly covered by Jane Mattes in *Single Mothers by Choice*. When dealing with what she terms "the Daddy Questions," she stresses how important it is to be comfortable with the issues so that "you can actually answer the questions very much in the same way you would answer any other important emotionally charged (but not devastating) question!"[4]

BECOMING A SINGLE MOM THROUGH DI

Some added challenges arise for a woman deciding to add a baby to her life when there's no partner to help. Choosing donor insemination, which is more controversial than adoption, takes courage and a determination to face any doubts, your own and society's. Single mothers by choice, or SMCs in the lingo of the national organization by that name, are women choosing to be mothers even if not exactly choosing to be single. The decision to head into motherhood rather than continuing to wait to find a mate has become a common one for women in their thirties and forties. The women who make this leap of faith in their family's future feel they have many strengths to draw on and much love to offer a child. But no matter how strong you are, it's frightening to buck conventional expectations of marriage before children. Jane Mattes didn't become a mom through DI, but her memories of the decision-making stage hold true for DI moms-to-be.

> When I first decided that I would have a baby as a single woman, I was so nervous about my decision that I had nightmares in which outraged people threw stones at me. In my slightly more realistic moments I simply feared that my career as a psychotherapist would be ruined . . . that my family would disown me or refuse to have anything to do with my child and me; and that my friends would refuse to support or help me and would respond to my times of distress by saying that I had chosen to do this alone and I had no right to then turn around and expect help from anyone.[5]

Many women write of comments from others that were definitely unsupportive. When you're vulnerable, it's hard to be the one doing the educating, but do realize your loved ones may simply know very little about DI and single motherhood and may fear the worst for you. Peggy openly shared her DI plans because she wanted to keep others from speculating if she became pregnant, but she also ended up hearing some unpleasant comments. She writes:

> One acquaintance said to me, "When your child asks where his father is, are you going to show him a piece of paper?" I responded that my child will only have a vague idea of what he's missing. My child will experience an intact family with one parent and one child as his frame of reference.

This tone, of confidence without counterattack, may help elicit support from loved ones. If you've met an SMC who's doing well, if you have a friend who has read lots and been enthusiastic, ask her to help you talk to your family or at least role-play such a talk with you beforehand. Lend family and friends your copies of reassuring books and articles.[6]

Many people assume single women will be open about the origins of their pregnancy, but, of course, many are not. No one has a right to expect a detailed explanation of your conception, and you may not wish to become the poster girl for donor insemination. If you wish to leave your child's origins a mystery for now or be open only with certain people, you need to practice discretion, because people will ask. Cheryl considered being mysterious but changed her mind.

> When I was planning to get pregnant by DI, I toyed with the idea of not telling people that I had had DI and just letting them think what they pleased. I'm really glad now that I was honest and open to questions because I think it helped the people in my life accept it and feel that there's no shame in it.

In addition to facing the reactions of others to your plans, you will be learning about your own responses. In "Maya's Story," Nina Shengold looks back on her DI experiences with humor and warmth, acknowledging that at first single motherhood "was like a one-way mirror. . . all I could see was my own doubts and fears staring back. I had no way of knowing that the world beyond the looking glass would be so fulfilling."[7] Peggy, too, is in touch with the losses but consoles herself with some benefits.

> As a single woman choosing DI to become pregnant, I have to face the loss of a partner to share in the excitement of the pregnancy. The labor companion I choose won't be as invested in the baby as the baby's father would be. I'll lose the typical experience of both parents planning the nursery and putting together the crib and buying things for the baby. . . . But on the positive side I can pick a name without having to compromise. I can decorate the nursery the way I want it to be. I also have total control over which donor I pick. Married women doing DI don't have this luxury.

Deciding to pursue motherhood doesn't always lead directly to DI. Jan recalls:

> When I turned thirty, I wanted to start a family. . . . I was actively pursuing single-parent adoption when one day a close friend of mine (a nurse) mentioned donor insemination. . . . My first reaction was "NO WAY!" . . . I thought about DI seriously for about one month (talking only with my friend) before scheduling an appointment to see the fertility specialist.

Many factors can influence the choice of DI over other possible pathways—a strong desire for pregnancy, finances ruling out adoption's costs, fear of custody battles if you conceive with a lover. Jan shares her deciding factors:

> Throughout the decision process I was dating one man. We'd been dating for at least five years and he wasn't ready for a marital commitment. I'd even approached him with the idea of having his baby (without marriage), but he'd have no part of it at the time. After I decided to go with DI, I told him and he agreed that I should do what was best for me. . . . Many things convinced me to go with DI. The fact that I'd carry and deliver the baby, the precautions taken with the donors, the cost, the convenience (I could do this at lunch break!), and the ongoing support from my friend.

Once you're ready to start, you may face a roller coaster of emotions. Nina Shengold found that the early diagnosis of some treatable fertility problems was frightening but helped end her early negative feelings. "Any self-pity I'd felt about having a baby alone was gone: I was thrilled to find out I could have one at all."[8] Peggy remembers her positive feelings during inseminations:

> I always believed as I was lying on the table waiting for the sperm to finish swimming up the tubes that I was instantly pregnant. . . . I don't think of the insemination as a medical procedure. I consider it my child's conception, and because of my attitude, I enjoy the experience. I consider it something beautiful. It's spiritual, full of hope and promise for the future.

But for many it can be a lonely time. It's sometimes hard to sit in the waiting room watching other women who have supportive husbands. If you aren't quickly pregnant, it can become difficult to manage your distress alone. Peggy, who also shared her Trying Times in chapter 5, writes:

> I'm jealous of my friends in Single Mothers by Choice (SMC). One conceived on her third intrauterine insemination (IUI). . . . I don't feel like I belong in that group. But the women in RESOLVE doing DI have different issues. Their children will have fathers. . . . That sperm to me

represents my child's biological father and may be the only father my child has unless I marry at some point. Most of all, it's difficult to remain hopeful.

Later her thoughts shift toward adoption and she writes, "I have no regrets. . . . If I don't conceive I'll move on, satisfied that I tried."

When women move on to adoption after donor insemination, there's a need for support, as hope and determination (and money) again need to be summoned for a new family-building approach. Many single adoptive moms can remember a time of great pain at DI's not working but are now very much at peace, even focused on the ways in which adoption is easier than DI. The pain of stopping treatment can be deeper for those who don't see adoption as their next step.[9]

For those newly pregnant, this time is seldom peaceful. There is a surge of joy and relief but also, at least occasionally, terror at the challenges ahead. Not only are they dealing with their own emotions, but they're also bouncing off the comments of others who hear their news. Jan recalls:

> I didn't dare talk with any family members about this until it was a done deal. Their reactions, I feared, wouldn't be positive. . . . I called my closest sister and told her the tale. She was surprised but supportive. I asked her to tell my mother before I got home. She agreed. I later got a call from my sister to tell me how it went. My other sisters were happy and very understanding. My mother was surprised but accepted it really well (considering she's a devout Catholic). My sister told me her first reaction was "Well, if anyone would do something like that it would be Jan." I was really shocked that she handled it so well (and very relieved).

As you become a mother, you'll probably get lots more support than you would have expected. Roberta says, "My family went crazy when I told them I was going to get pregnant. Once the baby was born, that's all it took to win them over." Anne Lamont, who wrote *Operating Instructions* about her son's first year, reports, "When women ask me how hard it is to do alone, I say, well, I haven't done it alone. . . . Sam and I are part of a great tribe—the people we love, who love us."[10] Support from SMC groups and friends helps. But the reality remains that you will need to draw on your own strengths and will often find you're on your own. Along with responsibilities, you'll find you have also added purpose and meaning to your daily life. Roberta writes:

> Everything I do feels better now that I'm a mom. It's like the missing piece of a puzzle in my life's struggle for satisfaction and meaning. Being a mother is an opportunity like no other. Lee's presence in my life has taught me so many things about what's important in life, given me thousands of moments to cherish, and given a love that's above all others. Having a DI child in today's world is easier than it used to be.

While many parenting tasks are harder for one, some DI issues may be easier. Talking about the donor seems easier, though still confusing. Roberta states:

> People say he looks much like me. I can see that now. When he was born his face was swollen, his lips huge, and my first thought was, "Oh, God, that must be what his father looks like . . . he was so ugly." What a risk to take, having a child with someone when you have no idea what his face looks like. That risk seems minor now. . . . Lee seems to me very much like the donor's description that I have in my safe desposit box. He's very athletic, loves music, very gregarious, loves basketball and baseball. It's as if my genes went on the outside and his biological father's genes went on the inside.

There may be a dad for your child someday. Having a baby via DI rules out only the most judgmental and conservative of men, probably not a terribly attractive group to you anyway. You will need to educate the new person in your child's life about DI. He will need to get up to speed because he probably knows little or nothing about DI. An open-minded man might react, "Great, no ex-husband to cause hassles!" If a man you meet would like to be involved in your child's life, there's no obstacle, even to adoption.

You may find that your feelings about dating and marriage change once your child is born. You'll be a family already, focused on your family's happiness, protective of your lifestyle. Sometimes the man in your life isn't someone new; he's someone now ready for family life. Jan reports:

> When my daughter was about ten months old, Dan and I got married and moved out of state. Dan was with me through the entire process, pregnancy and birth and raising a baby. He really seemed to enjoy her and finally came to a decision that we all could become a family. We don't talk much (if ever) about that time of indecision. Dan has adopted my daughter and we've since had a son together. Someday I suppose we'll discuss what he was feeling and does feel about not helping in creating our first child. I don't regret for one minute using DI, and I hope my daughter will understand how much I wanted her. . . . We haven't yet had to explain how it is that I knew Daddy before she was conceived and why he didn't want to be a part of it. I'd really like to find other children conceived through DI. I hope that she won't feel alone in this decision of mine.

Kids do seem remarkably able to deal with having a donor but not a dad. Their confidence may come from being so loved and wanted. Roberta tells of her son:

> The father issue is a big one in my life, but so far not in Lee's. We've talked about his father from the beginning, since I'm vehemently against keeping that secret or lying. And Lee seems to take it in his stride. His friends may ask, "Where's your Dad?" and he says simply, "I don't have one." Every time that happens I wonder if the circumstances of his birth will have long-range damaging effects on him, but so far so good. And I still hold out hope in finding that husband/father.

It's not always so easy. One SMC reports that her toughest moment was eleven o'clock one night when she heard her ten-year-old daughter crying. "I don't know who my father is." The mother told her, "I feel bad, too. I wish we could have a dad who loves us both."[11]

Your "tribe" of supporters may include other single mothers who can help you deal with the challenges as you fashion and fine-tune your responses to the wider world, especially as your child enters childcare programs and school, bringing new people into your family life. Single Mothers by Choice members have proposed a registry of families with the same donor. This has strong appeal for SMCs who sometimes feel their family is smaller than they'd like and their access to their anonymous donor too limited. But the term *sibling registry* can raise fears of unrealistic expectations. Irene puts it well:

> Knowing of one or two half-siblings would be reassuring/comforting, etc.; knowing about, meeting, becoming involved with several more would probazbly drive me crazy. I met someone at the SMC local meetings who was using the same donor as I was and I liked knowing that. I also happened to like her very much. If I didn't warm to the person, would I want her to know? Hard to say.[12]

Many will register in case young adults might someday benefit as they sort out the genetic influences of their donor. While this might or might not jell as a form of extended family, it can be comforting to know that possibility exists.

LESBIAN COUPLES CREATING FAMILIES THROUGH DI

DI for lesbian couples is simultaneously a pathway to parenthood and a public affirmation of their relationship. Taking this step is sometimes joyous, sometimes terrifying. Laura Benkov recalls:

> I was one of those women who with unwavering passion had always wanted to be a mother. In fact, that vision was the only part of my being that I knew to be continuous since the dawn of my consciousness. The desire was but heightened by falling in love. Making a family with my lover felt like the most natural thing in the world, yet it was unimaginable.

I knew no lesbian mothers, and the ones I had heard about had children from previous marriages. Though I didn't know it at the time, there were in fact many lesbians becoming parents. My lover and I must have passed some of them on the street as we walked arm-in-arm, imagining we were the only two lesbians in the world thinking about having children.[13]

April Martin writes:

As lesbian and gay cultures become more visible, the shame that results from secrecy and persecution is gradually fading. We have come to know that we are entitled to love and live as we want. . . . Having claimed our right to love, the next step for those of us who wanted it—claiming the right to fulfill our humanity as parents—was inevitable.[14]

Jackie had been with Joan for six years when she got to that point.

I had never envisioned myself bearing kids before this time, but I just felt like God spoke to me one day and said I was ready and now was the time. It wasn't like a burning bush or anything but instead a warm feeling full of support, hope, and light. It was glorious.

Deciding to move toward DI will require facing tough realities and powerful emotions early on. Lesbian parenting still brings out some homophobic prejudices in our society, even as the lesbian baby boom has brought greater awareness and acceptance.[15] The lack of legal clarity and societal protection for your family can make some early choices very difficult.

If you two have already found a supportive community in which it feels safe to be out, you may feel you already have the strong foundation that will carry you through DI decision making. You may be finding new joy in the opportunity to share a pregnancy. You may each be feeling ambivalence too. In *Never to be a Mother*, two women share their reasons for not pursuing pregnancy, including not being certain of their relationship's permanency and enjoying their freedom. Their concerns as lesbians per se were about negative societal reactions that might affect them or, worse yet, a child. Tina reveals:

I'm fortunate because my parents are very accepting of my being a lesbian, and they like and respect Gloria. Even so, when I mentioned my wish to have a child, they said, "Why would you want to do that to a child?" . . . It's hard enough for an adult to cope with being different.[16]

Many people presume lesbians have already learned to cope with being in a stigmatized minority group, so they'll easily take on DI's differences too. However, there are many shy, quiet, conventional, or private women who have until this stage been able to very discreetly keep their private lives private.[17] Mary and Sue told their story in *Parenting* when Andrew was five, but when he was conceived, they weren't out at all.

For the first seven years that they knew one another, Mary McFarland and Sue Buchholz never had to explain their relationship. When they were just two nurses living together . . . they simply went about their business and let people make whatever assumptions they wished. But when McFarland got pregnant . . . explanations were suddenly in order. . . . Until they started planning for pregnancy, neither . . . had even told her parents about her sexuality.[18]

The prospect of having a baby may feel like a goal worth facing homophobia. But it may feel overwhelming to add DI into the mix.

Two early choices for lesbian moms-to-be have legal ramifications: who will carry the pregnancy and how the donor will be chosen. If you're fortunate enough to live in a state in which the nonbiological parent can become a legal mom, and if you're comfortable with choosing an anonymous donor from a sperm bank, your legal issues in these areas can probably be addressed smoothly. But if you cannot both be legally guaranteed parenthood status, you face some issues. When you're starting a pregnancy, it's painful to have to discuss sad scenarios—what would happen if the biological mom died, if she couldn't provide health insurance, if your relationship ended. While a husband seeking DI knows he'll have paternity rights and responsibilities, legal rights aren't protected for moms-to-be not carrying the baby, nor are shared responsibilities guaranteed to biological moms. In *Children, Lesbians, and Men*, one woman says:

> The system doesn't recognize my partner as a mom, just because the baby didn't come from her egg. There have been court cases about visitation decided against lesbian mothers, because some guy wearing the robe as judge decided who was the parent, not by who was doing the parenting, but by biology. You better *believe* I'm nervous about the legal side of this.[19]

In some states, courageous women (and lawyers and support organizations) have won the legal protection of two moms for their children. Without positive precedent-setting cases in your state, you two need to locate a lawyer to help you draft an agreement of your co-parenting intentions. There will need to be provisions in the biological mom's will to reduce any chances of the co-parenting mom's losing custody to the deceased mom's relatives or to a known donor.[20] Meanwhile, guaranteed legal protections are long overdue. Laura Benkov puts it well:

> Wills can specify guardians, but they can also be contested. Parenting contracts are strongly recommended by legal experts, but as custody cases between lesbians have demonstrated, those contracts are often not given much weight in the courts. In other words, there is no adequate substitute for the basic legal recognition of family relationships.[21]

In *Family Values*, Phyllis Burke tells the moving story of fighting for that legal recognition.

> As the words came from the judge's mouth, it was like a dream. He was legally my son. I was legally his mother. . . . Should something happen to our Cheryl, no one could take him from me. I would not have been able to withstand the pain of losing him.[22]

Some women may attempt to gain both the legal designation of mother and the emotional experience of creating a child together by undergoing high-tech medical treatment. In an in vitro fertilization

(IVF) procedure, one woman's eggs are retrieved, fertilized with their chosen donor, and transferred to the uterus of the other. One couple, who already had the option of legal protection through a Massachusetts second-parent adoption, chose this procedure in order to share the pregnancy experience. As one of the moms-to-be said, "I want to carry my lover's baby!" If this sounds simple, you'll want to read not only chapter 5 but any book on IVF; it's expensive, with low odds of working without multiple tries. If you've settled in a state with absolutely no other way for both of you to gain legal status, this might be a wonderful test case—because a state with no other protections may simply repeat that old refrain "You can't have two moms" unless you take it to court.[23] To even think of anyone having to go to these medical lengths when legal recognition of your family life should be guaranteed may be infuriating. If IVF can advance to the point of less effort and risk with more success and insurance coverage, then this emotionally meaningful process may become much more feasible.

Legal shadows can also hover over your donor choice. It is legally safest for unmarried women to choose an anonymous donor who has surrendered all parental rights at a sperm bank. This can be distressing if you've felt it would be better to have a known donor. No one has yet studied how children feel about known vs. anonymous donors, but many moms assume known donors offer advantages when children later have questions. Lesbian couples were among the first to question DI practices offering little or no donor information and to request that banks set up identity-release options for donors willing to someday be contacted by adult children. In the 1980s many lesbians turned to friends or the nonbiological mom's brother for sperm. Some asked friends to act as intermediaries who would locate a man willing to donate without directly meeting the mother-to-be, transport specimens, and keep identities confidential until the adult child requested more information. This was also common then because doctor-controlled sperm banks often refused to provide lesbian women with access to anonymous donors. Now, as chapter 3 details, sperm bank innovations and infection risks make quarantined semen the usual choice. But some still wish to ask someone they know.

There are wonderful stories of known donors adding to the lives of lesbian moms and their children. In *Children, Lesbians, and Men*, written to support men donating but also full of advice for recipients, the experiences of families in touch with the Amherst, Massachusetts, Alternative Families Project are shared. One donor relates enthusiastically:

> I had a few good friends who were lesbian, and I realized that there were many lesbians who wanted to have children and their options were limited. I was not even sure if I ever wanted a child that was fully my own. The woman who asked me said she hoped the donor would be like an uncle. Fantastic! Imagine, being able to visit a kid and have fun with him or her and not have to worry about diapers and punishment and all that jazz.[24]

Even with a donor eager to help, there are worries for lesbian women who've asked someone they know to donate. It adds an edge of tension to even the best of relationships, and a falling-out with this man can have serious consequences. In a legal system that might view the donor's genetic relationship to the child as more "legitimate" than the nonbiological mom's, his later wish to expand his role in your child's life could be honored even if this wasn't your original agreement.

It can help to read many anecdotes about men's roles in the lives of the children they helped lesbian couples conceive.[25] It's wise to attend parents' meetings or join e-mail groups to learn from moms who have been there. Finding a balance between everyone's worst fears and most sincere hopes may be difficult. You'll need to become clear about the level of involvement that will work best for you, and then you can guide any possible donors and their loved ones in assessing if their intentions come close to your own. For safety's sake, we urge you to send your donor to a sperm bank to be screened and his specimens frozen just for your use.

Once you've picked your donor, you move on to the next chapter in your DI story, getting started with inseminations. Your decision about which one of you will become pregnant begins the lifelong challenge of balancing the roles of co-parents. Sometimes the choice is clear: one of you has always longed to be pregnant or is clearly more likely to be fertile. You may choose according to age, health insurance or leave options, or which one of you has the more accepting workplace.

That first month's insemination may bring some difficult or awkward moments as you learn to negotiate your way through a system designed to cater only to infertile couples. Jackie and Joan had found a local bank and chosen a donor, but picking up the sperm proved challenging.

> We were told by a "someone who knows" that if we gave any hint that we were lesbians, we'd be denied their semen. So I'd try not to look like a lesbian when I picked it up. . . . What a drag, being so in the closet for what I'd hoped would be an incredibly giving, loving, and hopeful experience. I felt like an impostor.

Fortunately most banks, including the one used by Jackie and Joan, are now more accepting of unmarried women, who are an increasingly large percentage of their customers. Infertility specialists and their staff may still be less attuned to lesbian couples. If you'd both like to share in your baby's conception, you may end up revealing heartfelt desires to some unwelcoming staff. Handling this may be practice for parenting, but at this vulnerable time of trying, an unsympathetic medical team can seem unbearable.[26] Gynecological problems or age factors may require that you overcome your reluctance. If you're starting with a specialist who hasn't yet worked with many lesbian couples, ask your favorite person on the medical team to be your contact person, at least until the rest of the team gets to know you. If you don't seem to need a specialist, do need to save money, and want to have a low-key, private beginning, you have the option to get some lessons in home insemination. This was the route Jackie and Joan chose.

> Our first try was in August and we used only one vial of sperm. It didn't take, but we didn't really expect it to. We simply wanted to do a sort of "dry run" to see how it would go and if we should make any modifications

for future inseminations. Joan, who's a nurse, did it herself with a flash-light, speculum, and syringe.

If you don't have Joan's skills or if you suspect any gynecological prob-lems might need to be checked, it may be wise to get some medical help optimizing your chances, because fewer cycles can save money too, as chapter 4 emphasizes.

Sometimes donor insemination doesn't quickly lead to a pregnancy. If you're trying at home, the pressure of worrying whether everything's OK can get to any couple. Jackie recalls:

> Insemination was extremely stressful. Joan and I fight and bicker a lot normally, but with this procedure we were neurotic. Did it spill? Lift your legs higher. You're hurting me. I can't hold twelve things in my hands! What a nightmare. Plus, it was all out of pocket at $125 per vial.

If you are using fresh sperm, you may be going to great lengths to inseminate month after month with your known donor. You may also fear over time that you're just taking too many risks using fresh sperm. Judith and Leslie had been very careful in getting testing for their donor, a straight, married, longtime monogamous friend. Still, his asymptomatic cytomegalovirus (CMV) infection, most likely acquired from one of his young children, was transmitted to Judith in the cycle in which she finally conceived. Not only did she have to terminate the pregnancy, but her immune system struggled to fight the infection for many months. By the time pregnancy attempts might have again been possible, Judith was approaching forty-four. She and Leslie did choose motherhood via adoption; they are now happily raising a toddler and about to adopt again.

Once you're new parents, there will be the usual challenges, such as getting some sleep. There will also be some decisions specific to DI, such as how public to be. Some women have gone wide open in order to make DI and lesbian motherhood more accepted and legally pro-tected. In their *Parenting* account of the reactions of loved ones to

Andrew's arrival via DI, Mary and Sue told of bringing her strict Southern Baptist parents to Andrew's dedication at their church, where their family's addition was celebrated.[27]

This level of openness isn't always easy, particularly for more private women. When Phyllis took over as at-home mom (because Cheryl was the legal mom and had to provide the health insurance to cover Jesse), she faced the stress of people's questions with her usual humor:

> Everything was fine as long as I stayed in the house. . . . People tend to speak to women with small babies. . . . I was not at all a public person. . . ."
> Does he look like his father?" "How should I know?"[28]

As time goes on, the comments and questions taper, but in the beginning you can feel like an ambassador to a not terribly sensitive wider world.

Kids seem to have an easier time than moms—or that wider world—in sorting out and accepting their family life.[29] Studies have shown that families with two moms function just as successfully as a mom-and-dad family,[30] and kids of the lesbian baby boom seem to take for granted that families are built in many different ways. Linda Saffron, author of *Challenging Conceptions*, devotes a chapter to anecdotes about children's responses to their DI conception and to their family structure, and these children offer words of wisdom and insight. Tim, twelve at the time he was interviewed, was very outspoken at school and even went on the BBC. These are his views on DI with two moms and no dad:

> Self-insemination is just about having a baby without having sex. What's the difference? . . . If people ask me what my dad does, I just have to say I'm not sure. . . . Sometimes I say I don't have a dad, but sometimes I say he's a lorry driver just to keep them happy.[31]

That kind of acceptance may grow out of lesbian moms' thorough preparation to answer children's questions with the help of books and groups.[32]

Moms do face "the Daddy questions." Interviewed in *Politics of the Heart*, Sarah tells of her daughter's confusion:

> We hang out with a heterosexual couple for whom the daddy is the main care giver. Whenever the girls are together, Megan starts saying, "Daddy, Daddy." It feels a little like a knife in my heart, but there are always going to be some drawbacks in an alternative family situation like this, and that's one of them.[33]

One little girl was much more perceptive.

> When my daughter was about two, there were three men in her life. One was her biological father, and he was the one who was least involved with her. . . . I'd never heard her say anything about a daddy, though she'd seen other kids' fathers in day care. One day she walked up to her father and asked him, "Are you my daddy?" He didn't know what to say, so he said yes. Later on that week I came across her several times singing, "I know who my daddy is. I know who my daddy is."[34]

Unfortunately, the wider world may not understand the lack of a dad—or to put it more positively, the presence of two moms. During the home study required before she could adopt her own son, Phyllis Burke received this "advice" from the assigned worker:

> She then fixated on questions about Jesse's donor and male role models. Father's Day would be coming the next month. . . . "I think you should have Jesse send a Father's Day card to the lawyer who has the donor's name and address, and ask him to send it on to him." I got a terrible headache. Jesse had no abandonment trauma. He had two parents, and he had always had two parents. His donor had been just that, a donor.[35]

Fortunately, these comments weren't made in front of her child. It's an added parenting challenge to fend off ignorance, about DI as well as about your family structure. But it's important to focus on the loving acceptance and joyful enthusiasm that also emerges. Jackie reports:

Almost everybody in my life was excited at our decision, friends and neighbors were thrilled and Joan was ecstatic. My parents, on the other hand, weren't so euphoric. . . . "This isn't something we know about. . . ." Translation: we're in our sixties and seventies and this is a concept that is so far out of left field we are flabbergasted. Then my mom just cried . . . . I think that my coming out was a complete shock. But to take it a step further and claim the right to motherhood along with this other thing that society so ultimately despises—I think they just couldn't envision putting the two together. . . . My mom finally did come around— from Minnesota, in fact, within a week of Garrett's birth. Over the course of my pregnancy she came to accept her new grandchild and rejoiced with me over milestones such as discovering his gender and feeling him kick in my belly. By the time Garrett was born, she was in "grandma mode." . . . My dad has never been comfortable with infants, but now that Garrett is two, he marvels at his grandson all of the time.

It's very hard work to get that little someone to marvel at. But moms say it's well worth the effort.[36]

The effort may involve even more complexities if one of you already has a child from an earlier relationship. A lesbian mom who's been through a divorce or the ending of another lesbian relationship so committed that they became co-parents may feel leery of starting over again. She may worry that her children will have difficulty adjusting not only to her new relationship but also to a new baby. Both moms and children may need some extra support.[37] Carmen was two when Joan met Jackie and had six years as their only child. Jackie writes:

Carmen was initially enthralled with Garrett. We call that the honey-moon period. Within three months she was realizing that this little screaming wretch of a brother was here to stay whether she liked it or not. . . . The crying, having to be quiet while he's napping, having a couple of moms running on too little sleep. I can't imagine because I am the youngest in my family, but for Carmen it was beginning to take its toll . . . [and] she decided to live at her father's house for longer stretches. . . . Carmen and I, sadly, grew distant.

If there's a stage of strained stepfamily relationships, lesbian moms may be even more anxious over custody and visitation. Fortunately, Jackie and Joan watched their situation with Carmen improve over time.

> Now, however, well over a year has passed and we are closer than we've ever been. I don't know if I just relaxed more and let her be free or if she started to grow up a little faster. . . . Her relationship with Garrett is beautiful . . . poor Garrett may have to deal with three mother issues (that Freudian thing). . . . She dotes on him like there's no tomorrow. As if giving Joan and me parenting lessons, she lectures us often on how we underdress him for the weather. . . . They play "big dog" and "little dog," racing around the house on riding toys, and they can cuddle and watch *Sesame Street* after a long day.

Most parents come to feel, surprisingly quickly, that the positive possibilities offered by their new child's influences on family life make all the added complications of parenthood via DI worthwhile.

While some couples are beginning their commitment to adding to their family, others are realizing their love relationship may not last, even though they have become co-parents with the help of DI. Lesbians ending their relationship must forge a healthy model of co-parenting without the divorce laws that would require them to hold to some minimum standards.[38]

Even if it might seem easier to walk away, your child needs to know you're forever bound together as his moms. In *Saturday Is Pattyday*, both moms set up their homes and their week so that Frankie can feel secure. "Only grown-ups get divorced. Not kids."[39] It can help to hear how others have successfully co-parented after ending their relationship.[40] As Toni puts it, "I live on a creative edge which celebrates a commitment born of love rather than biological imperative. . . . Kyla has never wanted for love from two devoted parents."[41]

Difference is a given for lesbian couples. No matter what your family structure or your approach to donor insemination, you can teach your children to cope with this. Raising children within a community that welcomes diversity is a lifelong legacy lesbian moms can offer their children.

WHEN STEPMOTHERS WANT A BABY TOO

When a new relationship brings stepparenting into a woman's life but she hasn't yet had children of her own, powerful emotions are often stirred up. She may not feel that her role as a stepmother is going to be fulfilling enough. But for a man who is already a dad, no matter how much joy or pain parenthood has brought the first time around, there may be little faith in the wisdom of further parenthood. While this section will refer to remarried couples, this is just as true for lesbian moms who are entering a new relationship with children from a previous one.

Donor insemination isn't likely to be an easy topic for you two to discuss. The motivation to add more children, at least when the efforts of DI must be involved, most often comes from the childless partner, the stepmom. The person already parenting may be altruistically concerned, may feel guilty, may feel it's only fair for his second wife to experience pregnancy, childbirth, and newborns. But there's also a strong dose of "been there, done that" and "been hurt already, no way again" for anyone whose first co-parenting relationship has already ended. Even couples who do share a positive vision of bringing a baby into their stepfamily may find the added challenges of DI a lot to juggle.

Books on stepfamilies seldom even mention donor insemination as a family-building alternative. This option's invisibility might make you think there aren't many remarried couples turning to DI. In fact, given difficulties with vasectomy reversals as well as the usual percentages of men with male infertility, many remarried couples do consider DI, although they often keep it very private. Outside their inner circle, many remarried couples say the husband was, however miraculously, able to start a second family. And few people suspect that it wasn't high-tech medicine or an expert vasectomy reversal that helped. There's some tendency to be more discreet because of the complex cast of characters, including an "ex" who might not be kind about DI and older children who might be confused or upset by it.

Deciding on DI may be toughest when the husband has had a vasectomy, as discussed in chapter 1. In his prior relationship, this dad decided he was done with parenting. His second wife is often distressed that his first wife was able to have his biological children, even more so if his ex pushed for the vasectomy that has caused all their troubles now. When first considering beginning a second family, they may have presumed medical advances would allow pregnancy to be a fairly straightforward, affordable project. It can be a shock to realize what efforts would be required for a genetically shared pregnancy.

Couples who consider DI after a vasectomy often worry about what they will say when people comment on their pregnancy. Many men were casually open at the time of their vasectomy, joking about doing their part with birth control or sharing their relief in moving on to another stage of life without babies. It's likely some friends or family members will wonder or ask questions if your wife becomes pregnant; certainly your ex will know you took some steps. Some men have felt foolish or disgusted at the thought of faking vasectomy reversal recovery or watching loved ones proclaim the surgeon a miracle worker. As with men whose infertility is widely known, these couples may feel they have to decide if they can be comfortable being open about DI or if they would prefer another approach to family building that seems less complicated to explain.

Male infertility in a second marriage sometimes presents similar issues with privacy. But often no one knows you are infertile, not even you, because in your first marriage, pregnancy began without dramatic efforts. Maybe the birth of your earlier child was a miracle or maybe your infertility developed more recently. Some conditions, such as varicoceles (varicose veins in the groin), can worsen over the years. If you're remarrying later in life, any chronic illness affecting fertility, such as diabetes, may have worsened.

A difference between couples with a male infertility diagnosis and couples affected by vasectomy is that health insurance might cover medical treatment for infertility but tends to discriminate against a chosen end to fertility. This is obviously distressing to stepmothers whose fertility prospects also end with his earlier choice of vasectomy. With insurance coverage, high-tech infertility treatment might allow hope of a genetically shared pregnancy. However, some who have tried many IVF cycles envy those without coverage, who felt more able to turn to DI.

A significant percentage of second wives want to keep their inner circle of DI confidants very small. There's a longing to have his youngest, most beloved, cutest child and to succeed in giving the "new" dad a happy home life. She doesn't want his second family negatively compared to his older children, and she may ask him to conceal DI from his children and ex-wife.

As is raised in chapter 2, DI isn't the pathway to resolution for everyone. If a couple can reach agreement on adding a child but differ on DI openness issues, it may be that adoption's greater social acceptability will be healthier for their family than either trying to keep DI a secret or being open. If they can't reach agreement on adding a child, she may reassess whether this relationship can work for her without one. He may have felt rejected in his earlier marriage and sense that this one, too, is in jeopardy. This will take time to resolve.

Some women are quite direct about going ahead with DI, with or without their husband's enthusiastic approval. A second wife may have lost hope for an intimate stepmothering role, or she may long to join in the lifestyle of friends who are now pregnant and parenting. She may have accomplished other life goals and now wants to add greater meaning to her life. Some husbands feel infuriated and betrayed, and some are ruefully accepting. Sandy writes:

> My husband had two previous wives and three children. I understood
> why he didn't want to start another family. . . . I decided at thirty-six and
> after five years of marriage that I really wanted to be a mother. Nothing
> could stop me. My husband realized my determination and decided I'd
> never be happy otherwise, so he might as well help.

She took a risk, but he shared her grief through the Trying Times that
finally led to joy in the birth of their daughter, conceived with both
DI and donated eggs.

If DI does look like a feasible route for you, it's important to
acknowledge the added challenges of stepfamily life. Yes, there are many
joys in adding a mutual child, no matter how that child arrives.[42] It may
take many years to actually become secure in the many roles and relationships you each juggle, but you need to work hard now to make
decisions that will work well for all the children in your life together. If
you're planning someday to be open with your child-to-be about DI,
you may feel that for now the details of his conception can be kept private until he can choose his own way through the stepfamily dynamics.

Stepmoms who have the prospect of pregnancy and motherhood
to sustain them may be able to make renewed efforts with their step-
children, who may need to know there will be enough love and attention to go around.[43] One teenage daughter wasn't at all pleased when
her stepmom, pregnant via DI after many months of trying, went into
labor on the same day her dad was supposed to take her for her driver's
license test. Yet the challenges of adding a new baby to a stepfamily
can well be worth every effort.

When DI Parents Don't Live Together Anymore

Anyone who ends the love relationship within which they began their
family with DI must deal with all the usual challenges of co-parenting
with an "ex" plus some twists. The percentage of relationships that

don't last lifelong are unfortunately very high, but of course, few men and women go into DI thinking their relationship might not make it. If the possibility of divorce were more acknowledged in society, it might be more customary for couples to outline plans for handling co-parenting topics that are likely to be even more divisive or painful after divorce, of which DI's disclosure is certainly one.

Unfortunately, any DI parenting challenges that arise after divorce may challenge all but the most resolved ex-spouses who have continued in agreement on how to handle DI's role in their family life. The lack of shared biological connection to a child too often is used as an excuse to sidestep the need to co-parent despite the end of a love relationship. The pain of communicating often keeps parents from handling DI challenges as a team. Whether or not a child knows of DI, she needs to know her parents' problems aren't her fault.

For couples who welcomed their child after a shared DI decision, there may be no doubts about continued co-parenting. Grace writes:

> When Evy was almost two, long-standing problems in my marriage finally became intolerable and I asked her father to leave. We are divorced. . . . We have joint legal custody. . . . The parenting issues so far (and I know that she's young yet) don't appear at all related to DI. . . . He's her father and that is that.

But for some couples, there just wasn't enough time together as parents to be quite so sure that DI makes no difference. Without the years of emotional bonding, it may be easier earlier on to think "not my kid" or "only my kid."

Some marriages do end soon after parenthood begins, especially if some aspect of the DI process damaged the relationship. Some men leave wives to avoid crushing losses, and this might be the case if the couple never acknowledged infertility's impact on both of them and rushed into DI as a way out of the pain.[44] One partner may have felt pressured into DI; the stereotype is that women pressure, but men can see DI as a way out of the unhappiness of their infertility. Parenthood may turn out to be incapable of saving the marriage. Sometimes a husband finally feels his wife is happy enough with a baby in her life to allow him to reveal his unhappiness. Sometimes both are aware their problems have come to a head and at some point agree that moving on with their lives separately is their only choice.

So divorcing couples remain joined not in marriage but in the responsibilities of co-parenting. A couple separating needs to focus on strengthening the bonds between the parent about to have less contact and the child, who usually faces the loss of daily time with Dad. Unless both parents are committed to maintaining the father's relationship with the child, the added complications of DI can lead to a father-child divorce too. One issue that must be worked out is communication about DI disclosure plans for the child. Many divorcing DI parents worry this information will someday be misused. Couples who had no plans to disclose may become anxious about that secret. This isn't as true for parents who have already been open with confidants and plan to talk with their child, but even these parents may now find it more difficult to iron out exactly when and how. You'll need to negotiate differences over DI disclosure just as you would have if you'd stayed married. If one of you now wants to tell your child of DI, the other should not presume that the message will be maliciously conveyed, for example, by Mom saying, "Your dad isn't really your dad" or Dad claiming, "I don't make time for visitation because I don't feel we have anything in common." There must be a positive message based on your child's needs. She will sense if one of you has made a unilateral decision and is running roughshod over the other's wishes, using her supposed "need to know" as an excuse to shift the balance of co-parenting rights, responsibilities, or power. Even if you haven't needed a family therapist or mediator to help you reach visitation and child support agreements, you may find you do need outside help to work out DI-related decisions.

If you've chosen to someday disclose DI to your child, he may at some point feel that his unorthodox origins led him to be unlovable by the departing parent or that his arrival broke up the family. Ideally, two cooperative parents will lay a groundwork that explains over time, at levels of complexity appropriate for the child's age, why you couldn't all continue to live together.[45] Whenever you do tell your child of her DI conception, whether before your relationship has ended or years later, she can then draw on an existing understanding that her presence didn't end the family's happiness. You also may need to help your child understand that having less time together can cause a feeling of distance more than any differences because of genes. If you can talk about your differences, you'll probably feel closer because of that sharing, and you'll be modeling that you're able to hear about your child's DI and divorce worries without feeling hopeless about keeping a loving connection going strong.

But if you let your child think DI is making it impossible for you to co-parent, it may take her much longer to recover from your damaging misinformation. If you two aren't totally committed to positive visitation or joint custody, your child may believe DI made for a weaker bond, when in fact other factors got in the way.[46]

If new love relationships begin after the divorce, newcomers must learn what DI does and doesn't change. Mom's new love may want to think Dad doesn't matter because he isn't the "real" father. Dad's new love may think he'll walk away from his child because there's no genetic tie. If your new relationships become ongoing, the partners need to understand that they'll be stepparents to a child created in love who happens not to have a genetic connection to both parents.

The adults need to get their roles straight because they can be confusing for kids. The adults may be overly focused on the fact that the divorced dad has no more biological connection to his child than the new stepfather who's trying to assume a place in the family. A dad may fear that his ex-wife or her new husband will use DI as a weapon to push him further away. Or he may use the presence of the new "dad" as a justification for walking away from a painful and confusing situation, particularly if he felt estranged even from the process of choosing

DI. Kids can sense subtle tensions, so you need to make extra efforts to offer them a model of positive possibilities, despite your own private fears.[47] The quality of your relationship with your child hinges on your efforts to deepen your child's bond with you and with your former spouse.

When Children Join the Family in Different Ways

Your family may include not only a child conceived via DI but older or younger children who joined the family via another pathway. Most resources on parenting siblings presume all of them arrived simply and in the same way. The term *blended family* was first used to refer to remarried families, but families involved with third-party reproduction bring even more complex mixes in which children can be genetically related to one, both, or neither parent.

Some people feel that differences in the origins and relatedness of children shouldn't matter. And in the majority of family activities and feelings, they don't. But parents who anticipate times when differences do matter may offer their children the best model of understanding their heritage and maintaining a secure place within their family. Before they can accomplish this, parents need to accept their own emotional reactions to differences.[48]

Parents often feel that it's important to be clear with others, and certainly with their children, that origins don't make a difference in loving their children. Martha Griffin, founder of RESOLVE's Massachusetts chapter, has often been asked if she loves the twin girls she birthed more than the son she adopted. Since they all arrived within one year, she jokes, "The one you love the most is the one who took the longest nap that day."

Many families blended through birth, adoption, and remarriage do include children conceived via DI, the oldest and simplest approach to collaborative reproduction. Because of the secrecy that has surrounded DI, many parents have never spoken about their feelings and perceptions of differences in their family.

Parenting two children with different origins does require more decision making. You may decide that you aren't yet convinced you'll ever disclose DI or other family-building issues you feel able to conceal, but even so, you must discuss this thoroughly as a couple to reach that decision. If you're going to tell your child someday of DI's role in his conception, you have to learn not only how to talk about DI at a level appropriate for his age, but also how to explain the similarity to or difference from your other child's entry into the family. Again, the secrecy that has surrounded DI makes it hard to learn from the input of others. Parents need to adapt relevant words of wisdom from resources on parenting after infertility, adoption, or remarriage. That's a time-consuming and often anxiety-arousing proposition. But when there are overt differences, when siblings compare themselves in ways that you know relate to their origins even if they're unaware of this, you can't really ignore deciding how to handle these issues.

Parents, children, and the wider world notice differences in appearance. When children join the family in two different ways (including via two different donors), the chances of significant appearance differences increase. Parents expect differences when adopting a child with a different ethnic or racial heritage, but unexpected differences can confuse parents, especially those who are unprepared to explain DI to a person commenting on characteristics such as eye color. Some families have complicated stories they couldn't possibly explain casually. Jim and Shelley receive lots of comments on Josh and Sam—almost all ravingly complimentary. But Josh doesn't look quite like Jim, who's his stepdad, and Sam doesn't really resemble either parent, since he arrived after an IVF cycle with both donated eggs and sperm. For people not part of their inner circle, it's often easier to let casual comments go.

As children get older, you may want to check with them afterward to see how they felt about a comment and what they thought about your response or their own. Kristi shares the story of Jamie's adjustment since the birth of his brother, Jacob, conceived via in vitro fertilization with ICSI, using Paul's sperm, a medical development not possible when Jamie was conceived via DI.

> Five months ago we gave birth to another beautiful baby boy. Jamie knows his story and Jacob's but he doesn't quite understand all the results. People started commenting on how Jacob looks just like my husband. Jamie then said he looked like Daddy too. I didn't want him to feel left out so we talked about the donor again. I reminded Jamie about how Daddy's seed didn't work so we got another man's seed and made him. So he doesn't look like Daddy, but he does look like Mommy. Jacob looks like Daddy because the doctors found a way to make Daddy's seed work. Jamie does a lot of things like Daddy, though, and has fun with him. Then Jamie asked, "Could we use another man's seed when we make our next baby, if Daddy's seed doesn't work?" As we talked a bit more about what it takes to make a baby, he added, "You forgot the most important thing, Mom!" With a bit of trepidation, I asked, "What?" "Love!" he replied.
>
> Jamie now mentions how he looks like me and Jacob looks like Daddy. He seems content and happy with that. We continue to just answer his questions honestly and I know he is growing up knowing that he is a chosen and loved child. He is very close to his dad now that the baby is born, and loves his brother, whom he prayed for.

Within the family, differences need to be celebrated as much as similarities. It's important to convey that sameness, in genes, talents, or interests, isn't required for loving and lifelong family connections. Even if you aren't dealing with the overt differences of adoption, even if you haven't yet disclosed to your child that his conception happened differently than his sibling's, you need to lay the groundwork that will help all your children someday be accepting of their origins. It can help to learn about many types of families with differences, not just the pattern in your own family.

Parents need to accept that they can't control what their children do with carefully presented information. There may be stages when one sibling tries to hurt the other. "Mom and Dad got stuck adopting you; they picked my donor." "Well at least my birth parents didn't go to some gross sperm bank!" A child conceived with the help of an anonymous donor may at some stage be upset if her sibling arrived via an open adoption and knows a great deal more about his genetic heritage. Helping her accept her own envy and express her sadness requires her parents to be very grounded in accepting the reality of those differences.[49]

Some families begin parenting via DI and then their second child arrives by a different route, whether a pregnancy with different eggs or sperm or by adoption. When a second pregnancy begins without donor sperm, you may feel some disloyalty or guilt toward your first child. In fact, only one of you may have even wanted to consider returning to treatment such as IVF with the husband's sperm. Women may feel defensive about wanting to carry their husband's child; men may feel ashamed about still wanting to see their own genes passed on. This isn't a rejection of DI or your first child's heritage. Many couples trying high-tech advances for a second pregnancy only do so with their child's donor specimens right in the lab as "backup" to fertilize her eggs if IVF doesn't go well with his sperm.

Even though your first child clearly knows she's loved, you could face some challenges. If you have had to try hard to get this second pregnancy started, your child might have picked up some of your anxiety. This may be your second round of the Trying Times, but it's your child's first. And if the birth is hitting at a vulnerable time in her development, you might be confused by your reactions to her sibling rivalry. You may feel protective of your new baby and impatient with her whiny behavior. You may fear these are signs that you love your second child more because of your shared genetic creation, or defensive if anyone else questions that.

If your second child is genetically related to both of you, you may feel less confident than before that you can disclose DI to your older child. You may fear he'll be envious of his sibling or see himself as less connected to his dad emotionally as well as genetically. You can avoid telling when your child is coping with added stresses, especially with his sibling. You may want to put some extra focus on sibling issues, reading the many books on creatively coping with sibling disputes and encouraging loving bonds.

Some families don't have two children conceived via DI because the wife now has fertility problems too. Parents may lose the comfort of her genetic relationship to their second child. But if the news of her infertility comes as they're discovering his fertility is more treatable now, they may face a surprising option, creating embryos with donated eggs, a second child with his genes but not hers. Gestational surrogacy might help their shared embryos survive, or they might turn to embryos created without genetic connection to either of them. Understanding all your options as an adult is sufficiently challenging, but your child needs your guidance too.[50]

When DI parents who have already learned to accept, even celebrate, different family-building alternatives adopt their second child, they may find adoption easier than it would have been when they were becoming first-time parents and easier than their medical options now. But adoption is much more public. Your second child will arrive without a preceding pregnancy, an event sure to capture neighborhood attention. There'll probably be questions about appearance differences between your children and about why you "had to" adopt. If male infertility has been a very private matter for you two, adoption's visibility may seem threatening.

If you have no plans to disclose DI to your first child, adoption may be a confusing contrast. Any discussion of differences related to your second child may raise anxieties that your first child's differences from dad might be noticed. It's important to work to get over that fear of DI being "discovered," as discussed in chapters 2 and 7. Your ability to freely discuss genetic influences and birth parents is important for the healthy self-concept of your second child. Fear of also dealing with these issues with your first child could create the kind of tension over family secrets that can be damaging for children.

If you haven't yet disclosed DI's role in your older child's conception, the adoption of his younger sibling may be the beginning of explaining that children can join families in different ways. Several children's books look at adopting siblings.[51] While you may be waiting until your older child is eight or ten to explain DI's role in reproduction, you'll want to explain the basics of adoption to her as you begin to consider this alternative. She can learn about birth parents and adoptees now and later be able to apply this to her own situation when learning of DI, as was true for Ashley in chapter 7.

Parents choosing DI as their pathway to a second child may be very new to the idea of family-building alternatives, or this may be old hat, contemplated in depth before they ever became first-time parents. If male infertility was diagnosed when you were still childless and then there was a miraculous genetically shared pregnancy or adoption, you may have already accepted that that particular miracle might not happen twice. DI can be a harder choice for parents who never knew they might have difficulty adding a second child to their family.

Parents often fear their second child could never be as wonderful as their first. And the drive to add a child may not be as strong, especially for dads, as it is for childless couples, who often feel they must consider any alternative. For those who still long to share the pregnancy and newborn experience, any DI doubts can be overcome.

Having a second child via DI is a common consideration for adoptive parents. Some didn't consider DI the first time because they didn't realize male infertility was so significant; they may not even have understood that DI might have been an alternative for them. Others considered or tried DI and at some point began to consider adoption as well. When it's time for a second child, DI can look even more feasible. The costs of a second adoption may be prohibitive. The couple may want another chance at sharing the pregnancy experience. Diana writes, "By this time expediency, ease and finances were more our concern than biology. . . . We had proof imbedded irrevocably in our hearts that blood ties had nothing to do with loving a child."

What to say in the wider world can be challenging. One of the most common infertility platitudes is "Adopt and then you'll get pregnant." So when adoptive parents announce a pregnancy, many people assume, "See, she finally relaxed!" Any plans for privacy may flash before your eyes as you long to retort, "Relaxation? Try donor selection and IUI!" Diana and Jeff had planned to be as open about DI as they were about adoption.

> At first we were quick to tell people about our daughter's adoption, but then I tried this approach with donor insemination. One day a neighbor who was herself an adoptee revealed . . . how hard it was for her to grow up with a sibling who was born to her adoptive parents. I offered that our daughter might not have such a struggle since her brother was "semi-adopted"—the product of donor sperm. The neighbor wasn't ready for such information and the shock registered on her face. I learned my lesson. I don't want to talk openly about my daughter's background and have my son feel his is unspeakable. So we are discreet about both and plan to follow our children's lead in whom they want to tell.

The differences parents feel about disclosing these family-building alternatives to their children can also be confusing. Parents often feel less trusting of public opinion on DI, so they can't foresee disclosing before their child could share in decisions about discretion. Nan explains:

> How we're handling the telling for each is very different. Our adopted daughter is five, and our other daughter is three. The biggest difference so far is the openness of adoption. It's just talked about more naturally. The five-year-old has always known she was adopted and that her sister was not. (She grew in her birth mother's tummy; our daughter by DI grew in mine.) DI hasn't been discussed at all. We don't need to talk about it for now, since the father's role in all of this hasn't come up. But

when it does, I know I'll be honest regarding the adoption and not about DI. I am hoping I'll be able to choose a time to discuss DI with my younger daughter while she's still young enough to make it her own without feeling we were dishonest, but old enough to have some understanding.

I guess my feeling about it is "gulp." I struggle with questions about the degree of significance in knowing your biological parents, particularly if not knowing your biological father is somehow less important than not knowing your biological mother. . . . I must admit that part of me would like to keep DI private; if we hadn't told as many people as we did, I would be much more tempted to consider it. But that would lead us back to honesty vs. secrets.

Some books on adoptive parenting briefly look at an adoptee's reactions to siblings later joining the family by birth. *Real Parents, Real Children*'s chapter on the preschool years normalizes negative reactions to the arrival of a younger sibling but looks at some added challenges if your older child is adopted.[52] It might seem logical to reassure older adopted children that siblings arrived in an unusual way too. But as Pat Johnston, the author and publisher of numerous books on infertility and adoption, puts it:

> One important thing to consider is what age-appropriate information, if any, the sibling should have concerning the conception of his sibling-to-be. In adoption it is usually advised that a child's personal information is his own, to be shared at his own discretion. If this is a transferable model, parents need to think carefully about whether or not an older child should have information about the younger sibling's donor conception or surrogate birth before the child himself does.[53]

Disclosing a sibling's DI conception to a young adoptee doesn't really help with issues of sibling rivalry and longing to also have grown in Mom's uterus.[54] But acknowledging upset feelings and affirming your love can be a tremendous help.

CELEBRATING DIFFERENCES

No matter how your family has formed, you want your children to feel confident and connected. You'll want to introduce them to positive images of family diversity early on. In *Families are Different*, Nico is struggling to accept looking different from her parents. Nico's adoptive mom tells her there are many different kinds of families, each glued together with love. Nico's conclusion reflects the security all parents wish for their children. "Now I don't think I'm strange at all. I'm just like everyone else . . . I'm different!"[55]

Chapter Nine

Guiding Those Who Care:
Advice for Confidants

Once we were pregnant, the first difficult question was whom to tell about donor insemination. We told all four parents, Heidi's sister and my brother and their spouses, and our closest friends, who would become our son's godparents. The reactions were mostly unsatisfying. My parents had somewhat shocked looks, no questions, no comments, no reactions. Although they rather awkwardly tried to be supportive, their reaction was to make sure DI never came up in conversation. Over the months I told each of my family members individually that we were comfortable talking about DI and they could ask questions. But few were ever raised. I had hoped they would talk about it with us and show that they were OK with it, but they were just too uncomfortable, which, of course, made us a bit uncomfortable as well.

The initial responses of our best friends and a few close relatives were more like "that's fine, who cares, it doesn't make a single bit of difference anyway." Even though we had sat them down and told them in a very serious way what DI was and how difficult it had been for us, they didn't get it. I know they meant well; they probably thought they were being supportive by minimizing what we were going through. But what they were doing was choosing not to share or even acknowledge the pain of our experience or our triumph in overcoming it. Although these initial awkward moments haven't damaged any of our relationships, I regret these "lost opportunities" for that bonding you can get by sharing and supporting someone in need.

—*Bob*

For better or worse, you've been picked as a confidant by someone who wants your support as he or she faces donor insemination's challenges. You may know almost nothing about DI, or you may know a great deal, and in either case you may feel uncertain how to meet the unique needs of the person or couple turning to you for support. Most DI parents are still quite private in the wider world, so support from the professionals, family, and friends who do know can be precious. We want to offer those of you who are new to DI the inside scoop. We hope also to deepen more experienced professionals' understanding of the complex reactions and varied responses that DI can elicit. We also want to guide professionals, organizations, and DI parents themselves to set up more support groups and specialized programs, because nothing beats the value of contact with others who have shared similar experiences.

FAMILY AND FRIENDS AS CONFIDANTS IN THE INNER CIRCLE

Throughout this book we've used the term *inner circle* to refer to the people in whom a couple has confided. This concept may become less important if DI is someday so widely accepted that people turning to it can easily be open. But for now, most people turning to DI are protective, both of themselves and even more so of their children. Those who pick an inner circle feel the need to have some confidants who do know there were added challenges in their efforts to become parents.

No matter how little you know about DI, you know your loved one has been through painful times—and that may make this even more difficult for you to handle. Michelle tells her story in her book,

Infertility: The Emotional Journey. "I know my parents care about me. I know they want to help—they just don't know how. They change the subject instead of letting me vent my grief."[1] You're already demonstrating your caring by reading this chapter. You need to be informed enough to be comfortable with DI before you can effectively offer support. DI isn't new, but this generation is the first to be more open about it.

It may be tough to read about DI families' needing support if you feel that you've already been insensitive. Since you probably knew nothing, or nothing positive, about DI, your first reaction can often be excused. Connie describes her mother-in-law's initial reaction:

> Stephen and I had discussed his infertility in great detail with his parents but didn't include them in our decision to use DI. They weren't asking, and I wasn't in a very sharing mood. Then I got pregnant. Stephen's mom was very happy for me. . . . Then when she and I were discussing pregnancy she asked, "How did you get pregnant?" Very carefully I replied, "We had help from someone else." She looked horrified. "You mean with another man's sperm?" Panic attack! Where was my husband? Why did she ask me when he wasn't there? I said, "Yes, I have an article you could read about it—would you like to see it?" I got up to show her the article from a women's magazine and then never went back to the table. I didn't know what to say to her. She must think I was a selfish, indecent person for using another man's sperm. I actually hid in the other room for the rest of the afternoon. . . . I never did show her the article.

If you have said anything you wish you could take back, your attempts now to understand why and how a couple is choosing to cope with DI, the healing passage of time, and any words of apology will help you all get beyond that.

You may be worried that you'll be relied on too heavily and get stuck in not knowing what to do. You may be relieved to learn that once DI parents have left behind the shock of the early months, when they first learned they'd need to turn to DI, and the stress of the Trying Times, they usually find DI is seldom on their minds. Once you are comfortable discussing DI, your job will be letting the topic recede.

Confidentiality is a major concern for DI parents, and you need to understand, early on, how they feel about this. You need to know whom else the couple has told and if it's OK for you discuss DI with any of those confidants. If you are the only one, you may feel trapped. They should presume you'll confide in your spouse, but what if you feel like you're lying to others? Even after reading about privacy in chapter 2 and elsewhere, you may feel burdened by this confidence, particularly if the inner circle is small or leaves you with no one to discuss *your* concerns with. The couple should realize that sometimes you'll need their ear. But could you also have one confidential supporter of your own? You can't suggest someone who thinks she needs to know all your business—that trait usually isn't linked with an ability to be discreet. Wesley had only told his immediate family, but his mom's best friend suspected something was up and angrily pried, as if his mom had no right to keep a secret from her. The ideal additions to the inner circle are people who can understand that the needs of the parents and child control how DI is disclosed, not their own needs to be privy to inside information.

When you have other confidants to talk with, you may not always like what you hear from them. Some may object to the way your loved one is handling DI, stating their opinion more bluntly than they would if speaking directly to the couple. You may be able to sort out these issues without involving the couple, especially if you feel the person is just venting. A more serious concern is realizing there's been a breach of confidentiality—or there's little or no respect for privacy at all. Then you do need to involve the couple so they can assess what impact this may have on their plans for disclosing DI.

Even when it's difficult to keep DI private, you must respect the couple's wishes and honor their choice of inner circle. Heidi's mother assumed it would be OK to tell her best friend; this news was passed on to her friend's daughter and back to Heidi. When confronted by

Heidi, her mother said, "Of course my best friend knows; she knows everything about me. I didn't know she would tell her daughter." You must be clear if you're entrusting information that remains yours—or your child's—to share.

Confidentiality can seem unfair, frustrating, or just plain silly if you think everyone is making much too big of a deal. But DI remains fascinating, a juicy bit of gossip to pass along. Understand that parents need privacy so they can lovingly disclose DI to their child when they feel the time is right.

What *can* you do to help? Try to get a sense of what kind of support the couple wants and needs. Obviously it's ideal to ask them. But here comes the next guideline—if possible, let the couple raise the topic unless you've been explicitly invited to bring up DI. Yes, you need some guidance in learning about DI—that may be how you got a copy of this book. You may have to be patient if no one is discussing DI. But if too much time passes, if you're distressed by their confiding about donor insemination but not following up with more discussion, ask the couple when would be a good time to talk. You may discover they were waiting for you to ask questions. After revealing how they conceived, Heidi never brought up the subject around Bob's brother because he seemed so uncomfortable talking about it. Her sister-in-law approached Heidi with some questions, saying she wasn't sure if Heidi and Bob were comfortable talking about DI. Heidi really appreciated the concern she showed and felt more comfortable with her questions than with his awkward silence.

Sometimes the biggest worries are over *what* to say. You can't be expected to know exactly the right thing, even if you've pored over this book. The right thing to say for one person may be wrong for another—even if they're married to each other. Robin writes, "My husband's aunt in the simplicity of her words 'I'm sorry' left us feeling so refreshed. We didn't have to answer questions or defend our position. We simply felt understood." Lisa's dad supported her by saying, "Any child produced would be loved unconditionally," which "really made me feel like we were doing the right thing."

If you put your foot in your mouth, don't take it too badly—the couple understands DI is an awkward topic. But if you insist on regularly saying the wrong thing, your loved one will get disgusted with your behavior. Don't follow in Helen's dad's footsteps.

> Before I told my parents how we conceived our children, my father decided to have a candid talk with me. He knew my husband had some problems but was sure medicine could "fix him." He told me not to pressure my husband because in time we would get pregnant. He then went on to say that at one time they thought he wouldn't be able to father his children, but the only other option was to use a donor and he would never consider such a repulsive option. If he couldn't have offspring of his own, he would only adopt.
>
> Later, when we decided to tell our parents, it took us a long time to decide if we should tell my father. When we did, he denied ever saying such a thing about donors. . . . Since then he's made it a point to mention the hard work it took to conceive me, since he had to "perform" sex on command. I think he does this to make sure I know he was virile. I have trouble understanding how he has no compassion for how his constant reminders of his own virility might feel to us.

If you are uncomfortable talking about DI, let the couple know you are and why. Anne and Clyde were deeply disappointed by some relatives' reactions, but at least she knew where they stood.

> They could not imagine we would be this "desperate" and seemed somewhat repelled by the thought of it. It will always hurt that I was not able to talk with my mother about something so important in my life, but she just did not understand and really chose not to be a part of our infertility issues.

If you have problems being supportive of DI, you may be able to reduce the hurt by acknowledging your distress and making it clear that you don't expect the couple to be swayed or feel responsible for taking care of your feelings. You may offer some hope that over time DI may feel less foreign to you. Or you may admit that you just can't imagine ever being a big supporter, which is wiser than avoiding the couple or walking out when DI is brought up. You're entitled to your own boundaries and may, at least for now, have to move to the periphery of the inner circle. If you can, urge them not to become discouraged and to reach out to someone else in the family or in their circle of friends.

If you have absolutely no trouble with DI, you could become the "answer person" for others who feel uncomfortable asking your loved one directly about DI. Abby's sister, a nurse, was designated as the person in the extended family who "knows all the details" and spared Abby and Ryan lots of stressful discussions.

In the years to come, what should you do if you hear of someone else who needs help with DI? You may want to reveal that someone close to you has also done DI. Don't violate anyone's privacy in your enthusiasm to help. Ask if and how they might want to be put in contact with each other. The mutual support may or may not be worth giving up privacy for the DI parents. The important thing to remember is the decision is up to them.

FAMILY CHALLENGES

There are added issues for parents of couples who are turning to DI. You may realize your child would welcome your approval, your blessing, no matter how clear they are that they'll make up their own minds. You may wonder if you have the right to express the full range of your feelings or doubts when they're in such pain. How this family crisis gets handled will reflect past communication and problem solving, but your child may be in much more pain than ever before. Your words of support, wisdom, and loving concern will go a long way, even last lifelong. So will any less wonderful words, of criticism, of disapproval. But if you walk on eggshells, your child will sense that tension too. Be honest, but use your best and most supportive communication skills in doing so. If it doesn't go well, be prepared to discuss how you all got off track, sincerely apologize for any damage done, and continue with further healing in the future, when everyone is in less acute pain.

The parents of a son facing DI may confront strong feelings. You may fear that something you did when your son was growing up caused his infertility. Some parents did get bad medical advice about undescended testicles, mumps, or chemotherapy, but often the result would have been the same no matter what medical care you'd found. Infertility is especially poignant for mothers of DES sons, who didn't know that the medicine they were taking to prevent miscarriage would hurt their child's chances of becoming a parent himself.

Parents may be surprised by their reactions when learning about DI. Your distress isn't only for your son's pain. You, too, are losing the genetic connection with your grandchildren. You may be sad that a grandchild won't look like your son, or feel confused about a nonbiological child carrying on the family name. You may fear your son will never get to experience the connection you have with him. You may envy your daughter-in-law's side of the family having genetic continuity. You may wonder if your daughter-in-law pressured your son into DI or openness. Maybe you wish you'd never been told, never had to struggle with these feelings. If your worries continue, your son may be able to guide you to others you can talk to—DI parents and grandparents, a DI support group leader, a RESOLVE phone contact.

The parents of a daughter carrying a DI baby also experience powerful feelings. You may feel sorry that she doesn't get to have a "normal" pregnancy. You may worry about the health risks of being inseminated. If you've ever had any doubts about your son-in-law, you may worry that he won't handle this well, even wonder why she's putting up with DI for him. If he's the best son-in-law you could imagine, you may feel protective, wish she'd adopt so he wouldn't be hurt by her "selfish" longing for a pregnancy. Some of the joy involved in being a grandparent is bragging about how cute or smart or just like your relatives your grandchildren are. Now you realize you'll need to be sensitive to the feelings of your son-in-law and his side of the family. It's great if you can set aside any worries and offer your support, as Mary's mom did.

> She calls our son the "miracle child" and says that he has made all of us—her own children and grandchildren—even more precious. Just the other day she asked if we'd do it again to have another child. To me that comment showed the ultimate in acceptance and love for us, our son, and any future children.

Marlene, a DI grandmother, wrote an article recalling her reactions after learning her daughter and son-in-law would need to consider DI.

> I wished I could help make everything OK like I used to kiss away your hurts. . . . Then you told me you were going to try donor insemination! I stayed calm on the phone but my head and heart recoiled at the news. . . . Why not adopt a child instead? There would be no swelling abdomen as a constant reminder of your husband's sterility; both of you would be starting parenthood equally. And how would friends and relatives react? Why not adopt and avoid all these problems and make life easier for everyone? But deep in my mother heart I knew why not. You needed, longed, craved to carry your child in your own body, not carry it away from someone else's. This mother finally realized your need to be a mother in the fullest sense. It was then that I rejoiced at this chance medical science was giving you and prayed that the treatments would work.[2]

Sisters and brothers are the relatives most expected to accept DI uncritically, with empathy and clearcut support. But of course, you may have the same range of objections to DI as anyone else. There may have already been tensions over a sibling's childlessness, and it's understandable if you resent his or her pain around pregnancies and children marring your family time. If may help if you can imagine how devastated you'd be if you couldn't have kids. Mary's brother's support was ideal.

> I confided in my older brother (who has three kids of his own) about my fears surrounding each of our child-creating choices. I'll never forget his

response: "However you have a child doesn't really matter. That child will always be accepted as a member of our family—as a niece, nephew, cousin and grandchild—just like my own kids."

You may feel hurt that your sibling expected any less of you. Grace and her husband waited until their baby was born so that first impressions wouldn't be affected by DI. Her sister didn't understand this rationale at first. Grace writes:

I assured them that it wasn't a matter of trust that they hadn't been told before, but just that we wanted them to meet our daughter before knowing that much about her. The silence was a little awkward before my sister said, "Well thanks for telling us . . . but actually, she's my niece. It doesn't matter to me how she got here, I'm just glad she's here."

If you are the brother of an infertile man and you don't yet have children, you may worry about having the same problem. And if you don't, you may be reading the sections about brothers donating sperm. Some brothers feel insulted if they're not asked to be the donor, while others fear they might be. Most infertile men dread telling other men because the response is often "joking" to break the tension, so for now, your willingness to listen is gift enough.

CHALLENGES FOR FRIENDS

Friends may have the toughest job in the inner circle. For some DI may be approached the same as any other major life challenge—your friend may just want some company and distraction from the pain. Don't hesitate to do the things you've always enjoyed together. If you hold the title of "best friend," expectations may be much higher. If you have children, you may already have sensed your friend's pain, especially during your pregnancy. Becki explains:

My friends try to be supportive, but most of them are pregnant or new mothers. I try to be happy for them, but they are so absorbed in their babies. It's not that they don't care about me, but they seem to be embarrassed to talk about it and afraid to bring it up. Nobody really asks how I'm doing or what they can do to help or at least make me feel better. Not that there's anything anyone can do.

It's also difficult if your mutual friends don't know about your friend's choice of DI. It's awkward when someone not in the know makes a comment that presumes everyone gets pregnant easily the old-fashioned way. Even if your friend can brush off such moments, you may need some help in feeling OK. You may feel guilty about not telling a mutual friend, especially if you think you could stop those awkward comments. Focus on helping your friend move through this crisis so that you can all get back to the more positive parts of your relationship.

If friends have also turned to DI, the support can be amazing. Connie and Stephen went to college with Carl and Louise, who later helped them move toward DI. Connie writes:

> That summer, just after finding out about the zero sperm count and before we had any answers, we visited friends who had been undergoing fertility treatments for years. They told us about RESOLVE, showed us the RESOLVE newsletters, and let us borrow them for a while. They told us about all of the avenues they had gone down, including using both his brother and anonymous donors to help in their endeavors to have a child. They told us about how wonderful their support group was and how it made them happy, even though they still had no child. . . . Actually, it was their stories that led us to our next steps. This was truly the beginning of the climb back to hope.

Rae and Bruce also turned to their circle of friends for help.

> We first heard about DI through a friend who had a friend who conceived this way. . . . The support we continue to get from our friends' friend has been very valuable to us. They are now pregnant with their second DI child and we continue to correspond and share our miracles.

If DI works, these issues will soon fade into the background. Your loved one will happily move on to parenting, where the big issues you'll discuss will be baby-sitting and birthday party plans!

ADVICE FOR MEDICAL AND SPERM BANK PROFESSIONALS

A couple using DI doesn't decide whether to confide in health care or sperm bank professionals; you're necessarily and immediately part of their inner circle. For many you are the only inner circle. Janet and Darren's urologist recommended a workshop for DI parents, but no one else in their "real life" knew. As they joked with the group, "DI has been a total secret—except for the twenty-one medical professionals who know!" The relief that you can offer with a sympathetic smile or phrase is magnified when a couple isn't confiding elsewhere.

This book teaches couples to work well with professionals. They may not have in-depth medical knowledge, but only they know their needs. We want to guide you in drawing out that knowledge—or at least not inadvertently setting up obstacles! And we want to make a plug for referring to, or even offering, services that can make the experience of DI not only medically but emotionally successful.

Your patients do need help with decision making. Kristi writes:

> I make decisions better if I can express them to somebody. And if you have doctors and nurses who will listen to you, it's really important to how you handle your whole infertility thing, the decision you finally make on what you're going to do as a family. You know they give you the information, but it's also the listening, helping you to think it out, especially for people who do not feel comfortable telling anybody else about their infertility.

You may want to pick someone on the medical team to keep a file on articles, books, and organizations of interest to DI families. Joining organizations like RESOLVE is a good step toward staying up-to-date on the latest resources—for you and your patients. Aline Zoldbrod, author of *Men, Women, and Infertility*, shares one DI patient's assessment.

> I suspect that it often takes a blow-up or tears before a doctor or nurse refers a patient to RESOLVE for support. Since it seems typical of infertiles to sit on such feelings for months or years, believing that "this month, we'll have a happy ending," I wish that RESOLVE were mentioned routinely on the first visit.[3]

You may hesitate to suggest a book, group, or service that might somehow distress your patient, but remember that the lack of any support is terribly distressing too. If you don't know much about a resource, acknowledge that to your patient. But don't let worry about imperfections keep you from letting your patients know that benefits might far outweigh any limitations. They are adults and can define what they do and don't want to follow through with. Heidi met a well-known doctor at a RESOLVE program; he had the courage to order fifty copies of this book for his DI patients before it was even written!

Peer support is something you can encourage without suggesting that a couple be widely open. In fact, providing a confidential way to reach others who have done DI may be the best way to give your patients a temporary support system until they can decide which relatives and friends could also offer support. You can ask your patients if they wish to be put in contact with other DI couples, either in your practice or through RESOLVE. At the very least, tell them stories of other families who have successfully dealt with DI; it's easy to keep out identifying details. You may find a peer contact person right in your practice, a service you can read about at the end of this chapter. Since many are reluctant to be too open locally, encourage patients to seek more national contacts. The Internet, for example, has become an amazing source of support that allows the option of confidentiality to your patients.

Privacy is also protected with counseling professionals. Doctors often refer to psychiatrists, relying on medical school training, but specialists in DI issues are likely to be psychologists and social workers. Try not to lock your practice into just one professional's vision of DI recovery.

Nowadays, medical teams and sperm bank staff face overlapping roles and shared challenges. In the fresh sperm days the medical team dealt with all aspects of DI, including donor screening and records, but now many people turn directly to the banks for information and support as well. The couple's medical team may or may not smoothly interface with their sperm bank. It isn't uncommon to have a doctor most comfortable with anonymous DI being asked by patients to work with a sperm bank offering identity release—or vice versa. We believe that fully informed consent requires that you explain not only how your system works but also what other resources exist. While there are business and competitive realities, the "product" of a child and a family at peace with DI is far too precious to present only your services and approaches. They will someday realize such options as identity release exist, so you may as well earn their trust by your objectivity.

We will continue out on this limb, and ask you to help your colleagues keep an open mind on the trend toward openness. A recent article found that one of the primary reasons parents were not disclosing DI was the lack of sufficient information about the donor.[4] You can prepare both donors and recipients now involved in DI to meet the needs children may someday have, such as corresponding through an intermediary.

If your involvement with DI goes back to fresh sperm days, you probably feel concerned or defensive about demands for openness. When DI was not at all legally protected or societally accepted, professionals never envisioned future requests from adult children. So now what do you do? If you're in touch with former donors, broach the topic and ask if they would considered releasing further information. Chapter 3 reviews research with donors, many of whom are willing to work through a trusted intermediary to answer questions that families might have, and some of whom are not opposed to face-to-face meetings. Xytex recently asked a long-retired donor to fill out the current long profile for a curious teen and his grateful parent. Re-create any records you can from memory. With modern advances in medicine, such as bone marrow transplantation, it's only a matter of time until your memory of which donor you matched with which couple may have life-saving implications (not only for the children conceived via DI, but also for the donor or his family).

The minimum standards are kindness and concern for the needs of the parents who did disclose DI and their children, who often feel their rights as adults have been violated. You will be in a bind, obviously, because you will also feel a commitment to any donors promised life-long anonymity. You can develop discreet approaches to contacting former donors to convey requests for further information. DI families do need to realize there will be financial costs associated with the process of locating donors. They need to understand that no approaches to contact are yet agreed upon in this field, so you will be cautious and may not be enthusiastic.

For current patients, both medical teams and sperm banks need caring staff sensitized to DI's challenges. Grace wrote of her connection with the office manager who helped her pick her donor. "I am still in touch with her, and she is the only person on the planet who knows what both of my daughter's biological parents look like." Sperm bank professionals, who seldom get to meet the parents-to-be in person, work hard to establish a relationship by phone.

We believe recipients should be urged to call banks directly for help with decisions such as donor selection. Taking calls from those considering or trying for a pregnancy via DI is a demanding customer service area. Among recipients there's often distrust of sperm banks or frustration with the limitations of anonymous DI. Some find the profile information disturbingly detailed, while others find it distressingly brief. When recipients ask endless or unanswerable questions, it's hard not to throw up your hands and decide that any attempts to communicate are hopeless. But hang in there. Many parents remember the kind or helpful things said to them by someone at their sperm bank or doctor's office—they're just too overwhelmed to write and let you know. And sometimes there are policies that don't warrant a thank-you note, that do need changing. In talking with recipients, you may identify innovative solutions to glitches in a rapidly changing field.

Advice for Counseling Professionals

Many couples, already feeling inadequate physically because they can't have a baby the "regular" way, seek out mental health professionals because they're finding themselves emotionally upset as well. They are adults in crisis, needing you to respect and support their ability to grieve, cope, and reach decisions. Many clients need to know you are not looking for pathology, that you'll focus on the normative feelings and issues triggered by DI.

Couples considering DI have a lot to process in the face of personal losses and couple tensions, so their current needs are often significant. Any article on infertility can outline an array of possible issues. Barbara Menning has brought widespread attention to treatment focused on loss and the stages of grieving.[5] Models based on coping with a chronic illness have been adapted;[6] Boston's Mind/Body Institute teaches techniques to reduce stress in infertile women, who were found to be as distressed as cancer or cardiac patients.[7] Aline Zoldbrod has applied both stress management and cognitive behavioral techniques to infertility.[8] Geri Ferber has applied self-in-relation theories, calling for approaches aimed at restoring empathic connection and confidence damaged by "the extreme emotional and physical demands of infertility and the complex medical, ethical and personal decisions that must be made."[9] The wisdom gathered by clinicians working with RESOLVE chapters and reproductive endocrinology teams nationwide can help guide you in adapting any clinical approach to the challenges of DI.

If you aren't a specialist in infertility counseling, don't lose your confidence and send a caller or client away. There may not be anyone more prepared in that person's locality or HMO network. If you are the long-term therapist of someone now encountering DI, you definitely want to sit tight and see how you can help. You should learn if there are any specialized resources in your region (people often drive a couple of hours for DI support groups or consultations). A consultation for your client with an infertility counselor might outline issues for ongoing work with you; audiotaping that session will allow your client to share that information with you. If your client won't go elsewhere even briefly (infertility patients are often pretty sick of professionals and appointments!), you might ask if you could seek out a confidential consultation so that you can better help him or her.

Even counselors with a strong interest in infertility may face challenges providing DI counseling. Your lack of knowledge in one area, your difficulty with one issue, doesn't rule out your ability to help—but you do want to acknowledge that limitation. If you hate keeping up with high-tech medicine, you may find it difficult to guide clients through the Trying Times. If you disapprove of anonymous DI, you may not keep up with sperm bank options and might not be fully informed about donor selection.

Whether or not you became specialized in infertility counseling after your own experience, as is often the case, you do need to take into account what family-building choices you made and how your clients might feel about them. Many therapists who are DI parents are deciding not to disclose DI to anyone else until their child is of an age to share in the decision to be widely open. Heidi has been in this situation, leading infertility support groups without disclosing details of her children's conception. If you experienced female infertility and DI wasn't an option for you, you may think you're off the hook—until a client wants to know if you would have used donated eggs. If you adopted or resolved to live without children, clients may be curious about why you ruled out third-party options. Clients may presume you have some biases that would affect your view of their choices.

Although most counselors try to take an impartial role in client decision making, your preferences can creep in. Heidi's counselor at the time of Bob's diagnosis clearly valued the pregnancy experience. Her response of "Don't worry, *you* could still have a baby" wasn't helpful to Heidi in her grief. Similarly, a proadoption bias can show. As one woman writes, "Our first appointment with a counselor involved her offering us the names of five attorneys who could get us a 'healthy, white newborn in twelve months for ten grand.'"

The most common bias that disturbs clients considering or parenting after DI is a pro-openness bias. Andrea Braverman, sharing her expertise in third-party reproduction, suggests questions therapists should ask themselves.

1. What role do you believe genetics plays in a person's personality, sense of humor, values, goals, etc.?

2. Are secrets necessarily "lethal"?

3. Do parents have a right to keep any information private?

4. Does a child have an inalienable right to know about his or her genetic origins?

5. Would you want to know if your parents used a gamete donor?

6. Can you live with a secret?

7. When is the parents' right to privacy superseded by a child's right to know?

8. Are feelings about disclosure or privacy entangled with the husband or wife recipient's feelings of shame or worthlessness?

9. How will the child's family and community react to the child's donor origins?[10]

Some infertility counselors face a moral dilemma in working with clients who aren't planning to tell their child about DI. If you have training as a family therapist, you may be as aware of the children yet to be born as you are of the family member(s) now present. You may have read the literature on family secrets and feel you must pass along that information to anyone considering DI. If you see yourself as an advocate for openness, if you've fought hard with medical professionals to reform DI, it may be very difficult to counsel clients who have no commitment to the values you uphold. Some therapists in private practice might decline to accept such a referral. But what if you consult for an infertility practice and are expected to see anyone beginning DI? What if the client established a relationship with you long before she got to DI? If you sense resistance to openness, we suggest you go no further than gentle urging toward eventual openness, especially if you have only a new relationship or evaluative role with a client. Parents-to-be deserve and expect information about both the pluses and minuses of openness and secrecy. If they find you helpful, they may stick around to adapt your information to their unique cast of characters and life circumstances.

Client self-determination is a core value for psychotherapists not because we are afraid to speak up but because this is necessary for change. Adults form their own opinions and will listen to others, especially about parenting, only when new or dissenting ideas are respectfully delivered. You may wonder if less directive approaches, as suggested in chapter 2, will guide parents to disclose DI. You may be concerned that our words leave room for parents to feel justified in envisioning a happy family in which there's no plan to disclose DI. We believe in keeping families supported and connected as they move toward the opportunities to disclose DI. If you take a hard stand and anger a DI couple, you may lose their interest in even considering your belief that openness must be the plan. Their plan as they walk away may be to never give another counselor a chance to judge them. Elizabeth recalls her disappointment with a social worker.

> She was very judgmental about pushing for openness. She used phrases like it was our responsibility to tell the child, it was his right to know his genetic heritage, etc. I felt she didn't take into account the context of the

individual circumstances of each couple. I also felt this social worker had her own agenda (advocating for information rights for DI kids) more than helping the couple find what agenda was right for them.

Most mental health professionals do lean toward telling children of their origin at some point. But what if the couple you counsel strongly believes that a well-kept secret without family tension will not be a problem in their child's life? You may want to ask them to at least keep an open mind and heart. Guide them to pick a donor whom they feel they could reveal if they later decide to. Asking them to continue to talk to each other and to reassess their plan periodically keeps them thinking and shows no disapproval.

Don't forget a basic counseling principle: start where the client is. Openness may not be the biggest stressor right now. Phil and Maria had worried that DI attempts would fail because of her infertility too. He resented the focus of the required visit with his in vitro fertilization team's clinician. "She got out this kids' book on how to tell your child about DI. I wanted to say, 'Hey, you get me a kid first and then tell me what you think about how I'm supposed to parent!'"

Counseling is not the only role in which you can help DI families. Your advocacy for clients with sperm banks and doctors can get results in meeting a reasonable but unusual request or clarifying a misunderstood policy. Your efforts may influence a doctor reluctant to work with lesbian couples or known donors, for example. Your program development and community organization skills can lead to group or peer support services. Once your efforts get things off the ground, your clients can benefit more than you ever would have expected.

Peer and Group Support

Sharing experiences with someone who has been there can be invaluable. DI secrecy has prevented that comfort for most families. But with some attention to privacy and confidentiality, you can help link DI folks, whether you're a professional setting up services or a parent want-ing to be sure no one else ever feels so alone.

The earliest opportunities for meeting others involved with DI were via RESOLVE and Single Mothers by Choice, with services from a national office as well as local chapters, and smaller groups for lesbian moms are scattered over the United States. RESOLVE, founded in 1973, adapted its DI services to then presumed need for confidential-ity, with a member-to-member contact system facilitated through the national office, so "pen pals" could reveal no more than first names, at least until a bond was established. More recently, contact people are as likely to give permission to release their phone number or address, and parent networks exist in some cities. In smaller chapters, it's at least possible to link two couples with male infertility within a support group exploring all family-building alternatives. Chapters also try to be sure that each year's programs include DI topics. Suzanne, living in a rural area, was just glad to be able to talk to other RESOLVE members.

> Although Mike and I are the only couple doing DI, it still is a tremen-dous help to connect with other people who are coping with infer-tility. . . . Many of the meetings are composed of women only—but my husband has been with me to every one, even though he is the only male there. I am very lucky and proud of him too.

Most RESOLVE services have reached people at the stage of consid-ering DI or during the Trying Times, but Single Mothers by Choice has been more successful at keeping parents actively involved. This may be because SMCs face more public and early parenting challenges, such as explaining why there's no daddy. Chapter meetings offer breakout groups for Thinkers, Tryers, and Parents.

Single Mothers by Choice originated the idea of a registry to allow parents, and later their children, to be listed by bank and donor number so that biological half siblings could someday meet; others doing DI are also welcome to register. While this may not offer DI children a sense of "family," it will offer them options to explore genetic influences shared from their donor's heritage. Meeting a half sibling may prove more appealing than meeting a donor, who is much older. For parents it is an innovative example of supporting DI families without even meeting. By registering your family, you're doing something concrete to improve the chances that DI children will have some recourse to learn more about their genetic history. It may someday give parents a mini-group of another family or two who have something quite unique in common.

One important type of DI support group would bring together children conceived by DI after they've been told of their conception. Meeting one another allows DI children to see that they're not "strange" and to share their feelings with peers in the same situation.

New organizations will bring new approaches to reaching DI families. They will also struggle to find volunteers and funds, not easy when members are very focused on beginning and raising a family. In Colorado one woman began the effort to form a national organization specifically for DI families. The Alliance for Donor Insemination Families may take up many pages in future books on DI, not just this mention of its beginnings. The InterNational Council on Infertility Information Dissemination (INCIID) is another organization that may someday link many DI families via the Internet. INCIID was founded by three women in 1994 as they realized how much information and support could reach infertile people via this new technology. Not everyone wants to reach so widely; starting a local discussion or play group helps too.

Any parent or professional wanting to set up programs wonders where to start. Few medical practices offer groups on DI or link patients with successful parents volunteering to help newcomers. Fears of liability for any negative outcomes of networking patients often keep a medical team from figuring out how to overcome obstacles. A parent or independent counselor can pick a location, do a flyer, and then hope the medical professionals post the flyer and pass along the news.

If you want programs widely attended, we can offer some ideas. A huge draw is having DI parents as co-leaders or panelists. If an organization or professional can do the advertising, you can help those parents avoid unnecessarily publicizing their names. Consider a broader topic, not just DI; you'll draw more people with an evening on male infertility, which people can attend without explicitly acknowledging interest in DI. Carol developed a workshop for her RESOLVE chapter, "Planning for the Final Year," looking at when enough is enough and preparing for terminating treatment. A panel and breakout groups on various family-building alternatives gives a couple a chance to experience the support of a group. In the Los Angeles area Carole LieberWilkins brought together families in which one or both of the parents were not biologically related to their child. Both the similar and the unique challenges for parents via adoption, DI, donor egg, and surrogacy may help mutual support thrive in a blended group.

Counselors offering small DI workshops are already equipped to handle inquiries and can offer a private session to anyone not sure about a group. An infertility counselor known to area medical teams can urge them to refer new members and can steer participants through difficult discussions.

There are many who would prefer to set up a peer support group without professional leadership. RESOLVE itself grew out of a group in which its founder was a member. Many such groups draw on models such as AA or women's consciousness-raising groups. Even peer groups need some leadership. Some guidelines will help you enjoy volunteer leadership over the long haul—which is the best way to ensure that your ideas will continue even when you are ready to pull back from the level of involvement needed in the early stages. First, wait until you're personally in good shape and have enough extra time and energy to focus on the needs of others. Or start with a modest goal of locating three or four others with whom you can work through DI's challenges before setting up more ambitious programs for others. Do get some others to help—a committee, however informal—so that everything doesn't fall on you. Together, form some realistic ideas of what you could feasibly offer: a monthly introductory meeting to anyone considering DI, a pot-luck for parents spring and fall, a drop-in group at the area doctor's office. Set up some basic boundaries: names and details can't be repeated outside the group; if you run into each other out shopping, be discreet; and so on. You don't have to reinvent the wheel—some of AA's model can be adapted, for example. Set up a system for tracking members—which needs to take confidentiality into account. Either pick a regular place and time, with one committee member showing up no matter how small the attendance, or set up a mailing list or phone chain for the "core group" who will want information on episodic meetings.

If you're contacting anyone involved in DI, keep privacy in mind. Be sure you have gotten to the parent. (Yes, one doctor's office gave the husband's father some sperm bank news!) If you leave a voice-mail message, don't mention DI or anything much at all when you're not sure who might be listening—the child not yet aware of DI or visiting relatives or the cleaning lady. A message such as "We're getting together on x date" can get the word out. Someone could volunteer to have a phone line with an outgoing message announcing activities so that anyone interested can check discreetly. If you mail reminders, be sure nothing on the envelope indicates the topic; even better, leave the information inside vague too. These days e-mail works well—if children or bosses don't wonder about the messages. These warnings may seem excessive, but they will allow more private folks to also feel welcome at your activities.

What actually happens when you get a group of people together? Connie writes:

> We talked about problems with medical insurance and finances, our experiences during the insemination, our experiences with the outside fertile world. There was no one else in the world who understood what I was going through the way the other women in this group did. When

one woman told us her sister-in-law had announced she was pregnant, I truly felt her pain. We were so connected, understood each other as though we had grown up together, yet none of us would have met each other if our husbands were fertile.

Marlene, a DI grandmother, attended a program her daughter was co-leading, and her outsider's view reflects amazement at how powerful group support can be.

> Now the speaker is relating an incident that brings a ripple of laughter and I marvel that these people can still laugh about such a painful topic. . . . The large group is broken into small discussion groups. . . . Conversations begin and personal lives, like paintings at the art gallery, are put on display for the rest to view. But the viewers here are not critics; they are supporters, encouragers, empathizers. I feel the tremendous bond among the infertile. . . . The meeting ends. There are still pockets of conversation here and there in the room. I sense newfound support, newfound hope, newfound information, and newfound connections.[11]

One program idea, asking everyone to invite their inner circle, can be transforming. Marlene, brave to attend as the only family member, reports:

> How could I not have understood the pain of her infertility until now? Did I have to be immersed in congregate pain before I could understand the depth of individual pain? . . . This evening has changed me; I will try to think before making insensitive remarks and offering glib solutions. . . . I could have supported you so much more, protected you from callous remarks, been your advocate. . . . I watch the individuals and couples leave and wonder what they will experience and endure in the week ahead. I pray that they are leaving with refreshed strength, courage, and hope and I bless them for opening my eyes to the pain of infertility.[12]

Groups can also share what they have learned more widely. Heidi and Bob's support group co-wrote an article for their chapter newsletter.

> In the group, we received our first opportunity to very openly share our emotions and acknowledge our concerns surrounding DI. During the 12 weeks of the group, we no longer had to keep our feelings cooped up inside. Not only were we discussing issues in the group, but the group provided the stimulus for us to discuss these issues with our spouses more openly at home. . . . Since each of the participants had different views and concerns, the group was at times quite emotional, and we all had our views challenged. . . . The group actually improved the quality of the medical care we were getting, since each doctor's procedures were quite different. With the knowledge we received from each other, we were able to discuss and question the procedures with our doctors much more intelligently. Through the work we all did together in the group, all of our outlooks have changed quite a bit.[13]

After experiencing group support, some people want to offer that reassurance to others. It's amazing to think that the pain you've struggled with could help someone else feel less alone and more confident of her ability to get through this crisis. Heidi started a DI help line through RESOLVE, reaching callers all over the New York metro area. Your willingness to spend even a few minutes, by phone or e-mail, can steer someone in the right direction. You'll occasionally need to set limits with difficult people,[14] but you can guide someone to resources offering more help.

When one member of a group becomes pregnant, it isn't always easy. For some, envy and pain get in the way of feeling connected. If you're the pregnant person, don't panic, and try not to feel too abandoned if your DI supporters aren't leaping up to help you adjust to a DI pregnancy. When Heidi and Bob were the first pregnant couple in their group, the theoretical became actual, and others vicariously shared their reactions. Your pregnancy can be a source of joy and hope. Carol's monthly Trying Times workshops went through a stretch when no one got pregnant, so when Kep finally did, she was like the team mascot. David started the ritual of sitting in her "magic spot" on the couch for good luck! But do try to be sensitive to participants' wishes in how they hear about pregnancies. Answering machine messages can help prepare members who fear surprises at meetings. Carlos, hearing via e-mail, voiced one theme: "I can't get enough hopeful stories and another DI child is always so comforting to hear about." Talk with DI friends about helping each other cope with pregnancy news.

MEDIA AWARENESS

If you've been supporting DI folks locally, you may want to spread the word. While some DI parents are willing to be interviewed for articles if pseudonyms are used, very few are willing to do television or radio, where privacy in the wider world ends. If you want to get your story out, decide on your boundaries. A writer will tell you her editor won't accept pseudonyms, but stick to your guns. Ask a writer or producer for information on their angle and who else they plan to interview; there can be warning signs that this is a story you don't want to help with. If you wish to keep some part of your story confidential, such as the terrible thing your mom said to you, explicitly state beforehand that you're speaking off the record. You can push for rights to see material on you before it's printed or aired, but this will be met with disbelief by most in the media. Greg and Susan weren't worried as a film crew from NBC News came into their home. But they were shocked when they watched Tom Brokaw's broadcast. The videotape showed Greg happily putting the boys to bed, but the voice-over wasn't so positive. Susan recently looked at the tape again.

> The piece was as insubstantial as I remembered, but it really didn't bother me emotionally any longer. However, the quote at the end remains impossible for me to excuse: "What Gregory and Susan do know is the children are hers, and Gregory is doing his best to make them his." My big beef is that under the guise of being magnanimous, he manages to completely misinterpret and demean Greg. . . . He bonded with them at the

moment of their birth as powerfully as if they were his offspring, and his relationship with them is as profound and loving. Of all people to be accused of needing to "try"! I think the guy meant well but had only thought about the issues in the most superficial, jejune way. . . . There are very few things in being a parent that you feel 100 percent good about—but I absolutely feel that way about not having a TV and about being open about DI!

Another disturbing TV technique is to put you on a panel of "guests" with the goal of provoking controversy by getting someone to question the way you did DI. You may end up looking naive, defensive, or infuriated if the focus of the show is on problems with anonymous donors, sperm bank scandals, or the like and you were just going on to share how happy your family is. The media thrives on sensationalism; try not to feed that appetite!

If you have media expertise, help arrange positive media attention. Volunteer as a media adviser to others offering programs for DI families. You may need to work behind the scenes, even anonymously, but you can help shift the portrayal of DI in a positive direction. One good show or article can serve as a model for future producers and editors who so often believe only controversy sells.

KEEP IT SIMPLE

Many people who want to support those involved with DI make the mistake of thinking too much about DI. It's different, it's misunderstood, but it really is as wonderful a way to form a family as any other. Don't expect you'll have to help with lots of problems. Sometimes DI families just want you to celebrate with them. Sometimes they just need your caring attention to affirm their success and pride in their family life. As Laney, whose oldest daughter joined their family with the help of her brother-in-law, writes:

It was like blazing a new track through unbroken snow. We were clear on our goal and had faith in ourselves, yet we did not want to do this in isolation. We found much needed support and assistance from a therapist and from very close friends. . . . We believe strongly in the support, the wisdom, and the somehow spiritual connection we received from our friendships as well as from our family, our selves, and our relationship with each other. Support and connection must be there.

Chapter Ten

Humor in Hindsight

Humor has certainly helped us through the issues of DI and it is still helping. Not a week goes by without someone commenting on how much the kids look like me. When they say how much the kids look like Bob, we both smile, our little "inside joke." Since Bob is a biologist, we always joke about him cloning the children in the lab. Even after people know of our children's conception, we expect that adding humor, and laughing about what we've been through, will give others the chance to see that we are OK with DI and they can be comfortable with it too.

—Heidi

Through all the losses, traumas, and frustrations of donor insemination, laughter can help. Often when you least expect it, you're rescued, at least for a time, by the lift of a good laugh. Sometimes you make yourself see the humor in a tough situation because you'd rather laugh than cry. Your humor can have a sarcastic edge, getting out anger. It can be a gentle and heartwarming reflection on a moment of connection or caring. All of the above can help when shared with someone else who's been there. These are definitely inside jokes. Some may wonder if it's proper to laugh over something so profound and painful. We can only echo this sentence: Sometimes laughter is the best medicine.

When you first realize DI is going to be your pathway to parenthood, it can sound pretty bizarre. And if you've been through infertility, the indignity of testing can bring some of the wildest stories. One man went to a new, state-of-the-art facility with collection rooms designed to signal the lab when a semen specimen needed prompt analysis. But the wires had been switched, and instead of a light flashing in the lab as he walked out, an alarm went off! Thomas swears that his semen analyses were scheduled only when the most gorgeous nurses were on duty. "I'd walk out with my little jar and say, 'Here are my three sperm—now you try to do something with them!'" Nicki knew Ron would be OK when he could go for a laugh—and some TLC.

> I remember one time, Ron was buying all sorts of things for his truck (lights, CD player, etc.). When I asked him how much he was spending and he told me, I got annoyed. I didn't think it was fair that he was spending all this money on himself and I told him so. He looked at me and said, "But I have no sperm." I couldn't say anything to that!

Talking with your inner circle can bring funny moments as confidants struggle to understand DI. Sitting down to talk with her family, Sarah and Andy decided to lead up to DI gradually by beginning with their infertility history. She remembers:

> The history ended with me saying there was only one way we'd be able to have a family comfortably without going into major debt and that was "donor insemination." There! I'd said it out loud! My mother said, "What's that?" That about put me under the table rather than have to repeat it. My father said to her, "That's using the sperm of another man to create a child." My mother started laughing and said, "That's fine. I was expecting you to ask me to carry your child for you—which I would've done!" My mother is fifty-two years old!

It's great if you can find other folks doing DI to share support and laughter. June met Abby in a RESOLVE group and they decided to bring Alan and Ryan to a workshop at Carol's. The guys decided that confidential groups should have a secret handshake or a secret sign of membership. And what better than the sign of the crooked sperm, a raised fist with a crooked little finger, discreetly flashed when fertile people aren't looking. Ryan also contributed to discussions on donor selection. Abby's family is brilliant, so he wanted an average donor, "without the dork gene." June recalls, "We really had fun! We feel guilty we had so much fun!"

Choosing DI will bring new medical stresses into your life. You'll pick up some new jargon, and redefine some old terms. Sandi Glahn's definitions are better than Webster's.

> INFERTILITY: 1. Process of proving that human conception can take place under conditions requiring even less privacy than panda matings. 2. Defined by some as the need to relax.

> INSEMINATION: Ability to join her eggs and his sperm while he and she are in different zip codes, countries, time zones, hemispheres.

> MOTHER'S DAY: Second Sunday in May, when perfume, candy, Hallmark cards, and nice dinners are delivered to friends, relatives, colleagues, neighbors, and acquaintances. Rates up there with Friday the 13th.

> ROLLER COASTER: Monthly cycle of hope and despair, which peaks in the middle and avalanches at the end.[1]

Once you get started, your monthly routines will include activities the general public can't imagine. Asking a brother or friend to be your donor can bring some logistical nightmares, only humorous much later. Marie writes:

> There was a time when I was pulled over by a state trooper for speeding (trying to make up time) to the doctor's office with a sperm sample at my side. I think the trooper let me go out of pity—as I just broke down and cried when he came up to my window. I explained to him I needed to rush to the doctors . . . due to the sensitivity of the sample . . . and here it is . . . (holding it up) and I'm sorry. He just looked at me and handed back my license, saying, "Go ahead." I'm sure that trooper had a story for his pals at the station that day. "Oh ya, you should have heard THIS woman's excuse."

Laney had even more pressure trying to coordinate her cycle with her brother-in-law's schedule, since airplanes were involved.

> He just happened to be flying in on the day that my egg cells were ready. At least the doctor said they were! Timing was of utmost importance and we had not a moment to waste. It's ironic. Dr. W. did all the testing, monitoring, prescribing, and even tacitly okayed my using my brother-in-law's fresh sperm that month. She fitted me with a cervical cap for the occasion, but wouldn't allow him to come to their office, which was right on our way home from the airport, to help us out with an insemination. Where would we go? We really shouldn't wait till we got home; besides, that might feel too weird since my husband couldn't get off work to join us! This was the only time I had done this with my husband's brother when my husband was not around, but there was not time to wait till he got off work or we were all together. So we used the fancy hotel lounge next to the terminal! We each ordered a draft at 1:00 P.M., not our usual style. He did fine, coming out of the men's room with the specimen cup in a brown bag. I was nervous about doing it myself in the restroom. I drew it up into the syringe, put it inside myself. That was right so far, but instead of gently pushing the syringe to insert the sperm, I gave it a real quick push, and it squirted out all over me and my clothing!

There are many frustrating, awkward moments at the doctor's office too. Clyde decided to break the tension by getting a laugh out of Anne. As he came out of the lab with the precious vial of "treated" sperm, he pretended to drop it. She recalls, "I watched in HORROR!" Then she laughed in relief. Ida didn't have her husband there for her event, which is the source of their later laughter. She writes:

> My husband always tried to come with me for inseminations. After our first child turned one, we decided to start again since it took us many cycles the first time. On our first try, my husband dropped off me and our daughter and went to park the car. It just so happened that the nurse was able to take me right away or I would have waited an hour. So there was my daughter playing on the floor with a nurse while I was being inseminated and my

husband was parking the car. By time he got in, the whole thing was over. To my surprise, I got pregnant that first time. Will DI ever become so relaxed in our family that I'll tell my older child that she was there when her sister was conceived but her father wasn't?

Some of the funniest stories are about transporting specimens from the sperm bank to the doctor. Lisa writes:

The very first time I went to pick up the tank with liquid nitro in it, it tipped over in my car as I was traveling down the freeway. There was nowhere to pull over and I was afraid to put my hand back there to upright the container. I had never dealt with this stuff before and I was totally freaked by this point. I didn't know whether to pull over and possibly get hit or drive like a bat out of hell to get to my destination. I chose the latter and everything turned out all right except for a frozen floor mat in my back seat. It looked like frozen smoke was coming out of my windows. From that time on, I wedged the canister in very tight behind the passenger seat.

Catherine's doctor didn't have weekend hours and so sent her off to do home insemination, but she'd need dry ice. She reports on her trip to Brookline Coal and Ice.

It was an amusing kind of place, though in my rush I couldn't sit around for too long and soak up the atmosphere. There were lots of burly men in T-shirts bearing ice blocks and heavy tools as I entered the premises. I hurried into the office with my wallet ready and was greeted by an elderly school-marm type lady who looked like she was right out of a fifties sit-com. "Can I help you, dear?" she asked, and I proceeded to order the prescribed dry ice. When she announced, "That will be $4.95," I turned over my five-dollar bill. Then came the unexpected question. "Now, is this for a school project?" I detected she was eagerly trying to give me a reduced rate, but I was totally thrown and had a hard time getting out the appropriate negative reply. My purposes were an awfully far cry from a school project. I finally got out some sort of no, decided (I think wisely) not to elaborate, and was on my way with the goods. . . .

It is now coming up on six years that I have been constantly awed by the beautiful daughter whom the dry ice and a medical team, to whom I am grateful beyond words, helped conceive. Could she really have come from that stuff stored temporarily in my refrigerator? Now that she's into school projects herself, I'm reminded of that helpful and well-intentioned woman behind the counter. As a parent now, I often wonder with amusement if there'll be a classroom activity I'll be asked to assist with that may send me off to seek my discount at Brookline Coal and Ice.

If your Trying Times drag on, the laughter and tears blur together. Wendy made her saga into a film, and her words alone don't do justice to the poignancy and zaniness of *Swim, Swim* . . . .

I start to take Clomiphene, a relatively mild fertility drug, and, thankfully, I experience no side effects, except maybe locking my girlfriend in the closet once a week if she forgets to vacuum her hair off the bathroom floor. Okay, a few mood swings. . . .

One cycle we do . . . regular old insemination at home in our own bed. It's amazing how the concept of "old-fashioned" changes the longer you're at this. Our at-home method makes us feel like pioneers in a covered wagon. . . . After almost dropping the jar of sperm on the floor into the waiting mouths of our dogs, we finally get it injected.[2]

Trying at the holidays can be especially tough. Irene decided to cheer up *Single Mothers by Choice* readers, and let us excerpt from her seasonal adaptation.

The Night Pre-Conception

Twas the night pre-conception and all through the house
Hoped a creature would be stirring—a child, not a mouse.
Ovulation was tested for three days with care
In hopes that dark blue in large box would show there. . .
For donor selection we probed many banks
Discussing the traits of anonymous "Hanks."

Brown eyes, curly hair, mother Russian, father Pole
Twenty pages of history but nothing of soul. . .
Yet a donor was chosen and shipped and thawed
Sperm washed and tested and proven unflawed. . .
The great office staff while depleting my wealth
Answered all I never learned in 9th grade girls' health. . .
And you'll hear me exclaim, as I make this solo flight
This was no "sperm of the moment decision," and I hope it is right!

Once you're parents, keeping your sense of humor through all the comments about your child is an art in itself. Karen writes:

> One day Joseph and I were walking through a local mall. Mae was about six months old and some lady came up to us and said that Mae looked just like her father. Joseph piped in with "She probably does!" Of course this went right over the lady's head, but Joe and I just smiled at each other.

As more families are open with young children, we'll hear more stories of the funny things they come up with. Jane Mattes, author of *Single Mothers by Choice*, tells of one single mom's parenting challenge.

> One of our SMC members told me that she wanted to disappear right into the ground one day when her daughter, age three and a half, proudly told everyone in the supermarket line, "My father was a 'semination donor.'" But instead, she smiled proudly at her daughter and said, "That's right!"[3]

Joanne overheard her son Ray talking with his preschool friends about having babies. They were debating if a recently married couple in their sixties could still have babies. Ray wisely offered, "I know, they just need some sperm!" Joanne was amazed that she wasn't really that nervous about what other adults might have overheard and wondered. She was just proud to see that Ray had understood their DI talks and was ready to recommend donor sperm to others in need!

We hope to encourage you to save and to share your stories of laughter as well as your stories of pain. When someday we revise *Helping the Stork*, adding the latest in medical miracles and parenting advice, we hope this will be one of our largest chapters. If you're now trying to start your family, it might be difficult to find *any* humor in your situation. Do remember that once you've got your baby in your arms, worries about whose genes he carries and memories of your painful Trying Times will surely begin to fade away. And when they do, you'll find yourself starting to laugh again, at aspects of your experience you'd previously thought were anything but humorous. A child's smile is the best medicine ever invented.

Resources

The organizations below all offer information and support to those involved with donor insemination. Our brief descriptions of their activities aren't meant to be inclusive; do contact them to learn more about their current services. Since most are small, volunteer-run groups or nonprofit organizations, including a self-addressed stamped envelope with your request for information can help them more rapidly meet your needs. For those that offer memberships or subscriptions to their newsletters, your support can help them keep reaching out to newcomers to DI.

Alliance for Donor Insemination Families
Susan Hollander, Ph.D., Executive Director
9678 E. Arapahoe Road, #143
Englewood, CO 80112-3703
303-220-8400
AllianceDI@aol.com
Organization offering information, support, and networking for DI families.

American Association of Tissue Banks (AATB)
Reproductive Council
1350 Beverly Road, Suite 220A
McLean, VA 22101
703-827-9582
703-356-2198 fax

AATB@AATB.org; http://www.AATB.org
Professional association for sperm banks, issuing regulations and accrediting banks; can provide information to consumers.

American Society for Reproductive Medicine (ASRM)
1209 Montgomery Highway
Birmingham, AL 35216-2809
205-978-5000
205-978-5005 fax
ASRM@ASRM.org; http://www.ASRM.org
Professional organization for physicians, nurses, laboratory personnel, and therapists specializing in infertility; can provide physician and sperm bank referrals and patient educational materials.

DC (Donor Conception) Network
Box 265
Sheffield, S3 7YX
England
020 8245 4369
w.merricks@appleonline.net; http://www.dcnetwork.org
Organization for anyone touched by donor conception, offering information and support; two members wrote the children's book My Story.

Donor Conception Support Group
P.O. Box 53
Georges Hall, NSW 2198
Australia
02-9724-1366 fax and phone
WarrenH@ozemail.com.au; http://www.ozemail.com.au/~warrenh
Organization offering support to DI families and advocating greater openness in DI.

Donor Offspring
c/o Bill Cordray
1415 Ramona Ave.
Salt Lake City, UT 84105-3707
BCor84@aol.com
Organization offering support to adults conceived via donor insemination and advocating greater openness.

Family Pride Coalition (formerly Gay & Lesbian Parents Coalition International)
Box 34337
San Diego, CA 92163-9935
619-296-0199, -0699 fax
National organization offering support, information, and advocacy for gay and lesbian parents and their children.

Infertility Awareness Association of Canada (IAAC)
396 Cooper Street, Suite 201
Ottawa, ON K1N 7B7
Canada
613-234-8585
613-234-7718 fax
800-263-2929 in Canada
IAAC@fox.nstn.ca; http://iaac.ca
National infertility organization offering information, support, and advocacy.

Infertility Connection
18604-61 Ave.
Edmonton, Alberta T6M 2B8
Canada
780-481-6618
piryll@oanet.com; http://fn2.freenet.edmonton.ab.ca/~rpape
Infertility organization with international DI connections via the Internet.

Infertility Network
160 Pickering Street
Toronto, ON M4E 3J7
Canada
416-691-3611
416-690-8051 fax
DianeAllen@compuserve.com; http://www.infertilitynetwork.org
National infertility organization with literature, tapes and programs on DI.

InterNational Council on Infertility Information Dissemination (INCIID)
P.O. Box 6836
Arlington, VA 22206
520-544-9548; 703-379-9178
703-379-1593 fax
information@inciid.org; http://www.inciid.org
Infertility organization offering information and support via the Internet.

National Spinal Cord Association

8701 Georgia Avenue, Suite 500
Silver Spring, MD 20910
800-962-9629
resource@spinalcord.org; http://www.spinalcord.org

New Reproductive Alternatives Society

641 Cadogan Street
Nanaimo, BC V9S 1T6
Canada
250-754-3900
spratten@nisa.net
Organization offering support and advocating greater openness in DI.

New York State Department of Health

Blood and Tissue Resources
Wadsworth Center
Empire State Plaza
Box 509
Albany, NY 12201-0509
518-485-5341
518-485-5342 fax
NYhealth@health.state.ny.us; http://www.health.state.ny.us
Strictest state regulatory organization, offering a list of banks nationwide licensed to ship frozen sperm to New York medical facilities.

Parents Via Sperm Donation Listserv (PFSD-L)
PVSD-L@surrogacy.org; http://www.surrogacy.com/online_support/
pvsd/
Listserv focused on DI issues.

RESOLVE, Inc.
1310 Broadway
Somerville, MA 02143
617-623-0744
617-623-0252 fax
RESOLVEinc@aol.com; http://www.resolve.org
*Infertility organization with chapters nationwide, offering information,
support, and advocacy; can refer to physicians nationwide.*

Single Mothers by Choice (SMC)
Jane Mattes, CSW, Executive Director
P.O. Box 1642
Gracie Square Station
New York, NY 10028
212-988-0993
mattes@pipeline.com; http//www.singlemothersbychoice.com
*Organization with chapters nationwide and a listserv, offering information
and support to unmarried women pursuing parenthood.*

Tapestry Books
P.O. Box 359
1 Country Club Drive
Ringoes, NJ 08551-0359
800-765-2367
Info@tapestrybooks.com; http://www.tapestrybooks.com
*Mail-order distribution company offering books focused on infertility and
family-building alternatives.*

Endnotes

For books and articles listed in the Bibliography, full citations appear here.

CHAPTER ONE

1. Anonymous, "Difficult Choice," p. 4.
2. Liebmann-Smith, p. 98.
3. See Nachtigall, Robert, et al., "The Effects of Gender-Specific Diagnosis on Men's and Women's Response to Infertility," *Fertility and Sterility* 57(1), January 1992, pp. 113–121.
4. Franz, p. 105.
5. Zoldbrod, *Men, Women and Infertility*.
6. Levin, Bob, "A Few Words About Adoption," *MacLean's*, May 30, 1994, p. 48. Reprinted with permission.
7. Fay, Fred, "Decades of Progress At Risk," *Spinal Cord Injury Life*, Summer 1995, p. 14.
8. Casady, Dan, et al., "Sexuality After Spinal Cord Injury," National Spinal Cord Injury Association, p. 3. Order: NSCIA (see Resources).
9. Bernstein, Anne, *Yours, Mine, and Ours.*
10. Abrams, p. 46.

CHAPTER TWO

1. May, pp. 65–68.
2. Glezerman, Marek, "Two Hundred and Seventy Cases of Artificial Donor Insemination: Management and Results," *Fertility and Sterility* 35(2), February 1981, p. 185.
3. Hancock, p. 1.

4. Swanson, Hollace, "Donor Anonymity in Artificial Insemination: Is It Still Necessary?" *Columbia Journal of Law and Social Problems* 27(1), 1993, p. 156.

5. Karow, p. 147.

6. Menning, p. 155.

7. Annas.

8. Imber-Black, p. 112.

9. Diamond.

10. Zoldbrod, *Men, Women and Infertility*, p. 109.

11. Daniels et al.

12. Baran and Pannor, p. 26.

13. Braverman and Corson, p. 547.

14. Orenstein.

15. Cobb, p. 85.

16. Brown.

17. Farrar, Erin, "Letters to the Editor," *New York Times Magazine*, July 9, 1995, p. 8.

18. Cottle, Thomas, *Children's Secrets* (Reading, MA: Addison Wesley, 1990), pp. 1–3.

19. Berry.

20. LieberWilkins audiotape.

21. Klock and Maier.

22. Anonymous, "Difficult Choice."

23. Klock et al., p. 480.

24. Anton, p. 157.

25. Alper, Laura, "Effective Communication Is Key When Couples Disagree," *RESOLVE National Newsletter* 20(1), Winter 1995, p. 5. Reprinted with permission, National RESOLVE.

26. Liebmann-Smith, p. 99.

27. Riordan, "The Threat of DI," p. 1.

28. See Burns, David, *Feeling Good* (New York: Signet, 1980).

29. Riordan, "The Threat of DI," p. 8.

30. Bombardieri, *The Baby Decision*, p. 94.

31. Braverman, Andrea, "Egg Donation: Psychological and Counseling Issues Surrounding Disclosure versus Privacy," in *Family Building Through Egg and Sperm Donation: Medical, Legal, and Ethical Issues*, ed. Machelle Seibel and Susan Crockin (Sudbury, MA: Jones and Bartlett Pub., 1996), p. 281.

32. Golombok et al., p. 296.

33. Bombardieri, "Childfree Decision-making," p. 1.

34. Bombardieri, *The Baby Decision*, pp. 6–7.

35. Schover et al.

36. Klock and Maier.

37. Hanson, p. 104.

CHAPTER THREE

1. May; Marsh and Ronner; Pfeffer.
2. Duka and DeCherney, pp. 63–65.
3. Annas.
4. Bunge, R. G., and J. K. Sherman, "Fertilizing Capacity of Frozen Human Sperm," *Nature* 172, 1953, p. 627.
5. May's chapter on eugenics movement.
6. Drexler, p. 9.
7. Gill; Noble, pp. 117–121.
8. Sperm banks tracked specimens and later documented cases of HIV transmission before tests were available; see Guinan.
9. AFS, now American Society for Reproductive Medicine, periodically updates their guidelines for DI. Most recent: American Fertility Society, "Guidelines for Gamete Donation," *Fertility and Sterility* 59(2), Supplement 1, February 1993, pp. S1–9. Order: ASRM (see Resources).
10. Seligson, p. 38.
11. Ex., Chauhan, Mayursingh, et al., "Screening for Cytomegalovirus Antibody in a Donor Insemination Program: Difficulties in Implementing the American Fertility Society Guidelines," *Fertility and Sterility* 51(5), May 1989, pp. 901–902.
12. Carey, p. 56.
13. Barratt, Christopher, et al., "Donor Insemination: A Look to the Future," *Fertility and Sterility* 54(3), September 1990, pp. 375–387; Johnston, Robyn, et al., "Correlation of Semen Variables and Pregnancy Rates for Donor Insemination: A 15-Year Retrospective," *Fertility and Sterility* 61(2), February 1994, pp. 355–359.
14. Daniels and Lewis, "Donor Insemination."
15. Daniels, "Semen Donors," p. 124.
16. Fried, p. 111.
17. Cooper and Glazer, *Beyond Infertility*, pp. 184–185, 190.
18. Daniels, "Semen Donors," p. 124.
19. Mahlstedt and Probasco, p. 751.
20. Abrams, p. 49.
21. Drexler, p. 9.
22. Anonymous, "Confessions of a Sperm Donor," p. 154.
23. Abrams, p. 49.
24. Ibid.
25. Mahlstedt and Probasco.
26. Lobenstine, p. 12.
27. Seligson, p. 30.
28. Anonymous, "Confessions of a Sperm Donor," p. 180.
29. Mahlstedt and Probasco, p. 750.

30. Daniels, "Semen Donors," pp. 124–125.

31. Orenstein, p. 58.

32. Braverman and Corson, p. 545.

33. Philipp, Elliot, *Overcoming Childlessness* (New York: Taplinger, 1975), p. 121.

34. Blanchard, "Donor Insemination," p. 10.

35. Cooper and Glazer, *Beyond Infertility*, p. 157.

36. Lobenstine.

37. Nelson, pp. 142–143.

38. Riordan, p. 8.

39. McDaniel, p. 303.

Chapter Four

1. Menning, *Infertility,* p. 155.

2. Matorras, Roberto, et al., "Intrauterine Insemination with Frozen Sperm Increases Pregnancy Rates in Donor Insemination Cycles under Gonadotropin Stimulation," *Fertility and Sterility* 65(3), March 1996, pp. 620–625; Patton, Phillip, et al., "Intrauterine Insemination Outperforms Intracervical Insemination in a Randomized, Controlled Study with Frozen, Donor Semen," *Fertility and Sterility* 57(3), March 1992, pp. 559–564; Byrd, William, et al., "A Prospective Randomized Study of Pregnancy Rates Following Intrauterine and Intracervical Insemination Using Frozen Donor sperm," *Fertility and Sterility* 53(3), March 1990, pp. 521–527; Williams, Daniel, et al., "Does Intrauterine Insemination Offer an Advantage to Cervical Cap Insemination in a DI Program?" *Fertility and Sterility* 63(2), February 1995, pp. 295–298.

3. Byrd et al., "A Prospective Randomized Study," p. 526.

4. Shelden, R., et al., "IUI-Ready vs. Local IUI Processing for Frozen Donor Sperm," 1995 Abstracts from American Society for Reproductive Medicine, October 7–12, 1995, Annual Meeting, p. S254.

5. Franz, p. 106.

6. Sege, Irene, "Facing Life Without Children," *Boston Globe, Living/Arts,* October 25, 1994, p. 67.

7. Liebman-Smith, p. 141.

8. Ibid., p. 142.

Chapter Five

1. Schwartz, D., and M. J. Mayaux, "Female Fecundity as a Function of Age," *New England Journal of Medicine* 306(7), February 18, 1982, pp. 404–406; for 2,000 women using frozen sperm, fertility dropped after age 30 and again after 35.

2. Byrd, William, et al., "Intrauterine Insemination with Frozen Donor Sperm: a Prospective Randomized Trial Comparing Three Different Sperm Preparation Techniques," *Fertility and Sterility* 62(4), October 1994, p. 850.

3. Shapiro, Sander, pp. 469–485. Reviews studies.

4. Byrd, et al., "A Prospective Randomized Study," pp. 521–527.

5. Brook, Philip, et al., "The More Accurate Timing of Insemination with Regard to Ovulation Does Not Create a Significant Improvement in Pregnancy Rates in a Donor Insemination Program," *Fertility and Sterility* 61(2), February 1994, pp. 308–313.

6. Byrd, et al., "A Prospective Randomized Study," p. 525.

7. Brown, Cheryl, et al., "Improved Cryopreserved Semen Fecundability in an Alternating Fresh-Frozen Artificial Insemination Program," *Fertility and Sterility* 50(5), November 1988, pp. 825–827.

8. Carey, p. 55.

9. Silverberg, Kaylen, et al., "A Prospective, Randomized Trial Comparing Two Different Intrauterine Insemination Regimens in Controlled Ovarian Hyperstimulation Cycles," *Fertility and Sterility* 57(2), February 1992, pp. 357–361; Centola, Grace, et al., "Pregnancy Rates after Double versus Single Insemination with Frozen Donor Sperm," *Fertility and Sterility* 54(6), December 1990, pp. 1089–1092; Byrd et al., "A Prospective Randomized Study."

10. Rauch, Karen, "Keep Trying . . . ," Letter to the Editor, *RESOLVE National Newsletter* 13(5), December 1988, p. 2.

11. Zolbrod, *Getting Around the Boulder in the Road*, p. 22.

12. Anton; Lang; Carter, Michael and Jean, *Sweet Grapes* (Indianapolis: Perspectives Press, 1989).

Chapter Six

1. Glazer, p. 13.

2. Anonymous, "Difficult Choice," pp. 6–7.

Chapter Seven

1. Oldham, John, and Lois Morris, *The New Personality Self-Portrait* (New York: Bantam Books, 1995), pp. 395–396.

2. Bombardieri, Merle, "Coping with the Stress of Infertility," RESOLVE fact sheet, pp. 7–8.

3. Simons; Rosenberg and Epstein, pp. 260–289.

4. Schmidt.

5. Riordan, Tom, "Article Review," *RESOLVE of NYC Newsletter*, September 1995, p. 3. Reprinted with permission.

6. Melina; LieberWilkins.

7. Baran and Pannor; Probasco.

8. Zoldbrod, *Men, Women and Infertility*, pp. 103–104.

9. Diamond, p. 11.

10. Bernstein, *Flight of the Stork*.

11. Bernstein, *Flight of the Stork*; Melina.

12. Blau, Melinda, "Mommy, Where Did I Come From?" *Child*, April 1995, p. 85.

13. Noble, pp. 336–337.

14. Melina, pp. 92–97.

15. Bernstein, *Flight of the Stork*.

16. New South Wales Infertility Social Workers Group.

17. Infertility Research Trust.

18. Gordon.

19. Wickham.

20. Pellegrini; Simon; Tax.

21. Cannon, Janell, *Stellaluna* (San Diego, CA: Harcourt, Brace & Co., 1993); Carrier, Lark, *A Perfect Spring* (Saxonville, MA: Picture Book Studio, 1990); Schaffer, Libor, *Arthur Sets Sail* (New York: North-South Books, 1987).

22. Blaustein, Muriel, *Play Ball, Zachary!* (New York: Harper & Row, 1988).

23. Carlson, Nancy, *I Like Me!* (New York: Puffin Books, 1988); Modesitt, Jeanne, *Mama, If You Had a Wish* (New York: Green Tiger Press, 1993).

24. McPhail, David, *Emma's Pet* (New York: E. P. Dutton, 1985); Stephenson, James, *I Meant to Tell You* (New York: Greenwillow Books, 1996); Porter-Gaylord, Laurel, *I Love My Daddy Because* (New York: Dutton Children's Books, 1991).

25. Orenstein, p. 58.

26. Berry.

27. Schnitter.

28. Schaffer.

29. Mason.

30. Baran and Pannor; Cobb; Hancock; Roman.

31. Orenstein.

32. Riordan, "Article Review."

33. Seligson, p. 30.

34. See Resources listing for Donor Offspring.

35. Topp, pp. 149–151.

36. Hochman, Gloria, "The New Facts of Life," *Philadelphia Inquirer*, July 17, 1994, p. 27.

37. Brown.

CHAPTER EIGHT

1. McCartney, Cheryl, "Decision by Single Women to Conceive by Artificial Donor Insemination," *Journal of Psychosomatic Obstetrics and Gynecology* 4(4), December 1985, p. 321.

2. Benkov, p. 116.

3. Pies, Cheri, *Considering Parenthood*, 2nd ed. (Minneapolis: Spinsters Ink, 1988); Benkov; Martin; Mattes.

4. Mattes, p. 129.

5. Mattes, p. xvii.

6. Mattes; also Alexander, Shoshana, *In Praise of Single Parents* (Boston: Houghton Mifflin, 1994); Merritt, Sharyne, and Linda Steiner, *And Baby Makes Two* (New York: Franklin Watts, 1984).

7. Shengold, Nina, p. 103.

8. Ibid., p. 144.

9. Anton, pp. 24–25.

10. Lamott, Anne, "When Going It Alone Turns Out to Be Not So Alone at All," *The New York Times*, August 5, 1993, p. C1.

11. Lawson, Carol, p. C1.

12. Mattes, Jane, "Sibling Registry for Children Conceived By Anonymous Donor Is On Its Way," *Single Mothers by Choice Newsletter* 54, September 1995, p. 1.

13. Benkov, p. 3.

14. Martin, p. 6.

15. Kantrowitz, Barbara, "Gay Families Come Out," *Newsweek* 28(19), November 4, 1996, pp. 50–57.

16. Anton, pp. 52–56.

17. Lowell, Jax Peters, *Mothers* (New York: St. Martin's Griffin, 1996). Powerful fiction.

18. Clendinen, Dudley, "My Two Moms," *Parenting*, March 1995, p. 100.

19. Lobenstine, p. 30.

20. Schwab, Rochelle Hollander, *In a Family Way* (Alexandria, VA: Orlando Place Press, 1995).(Fiction from P-FLAG mom; order: 3617 Orlando Place, Alexandria, VA 22305, $10.95.)

21. Benkov, p. 249.

22. Burke, Phyllis, *Family Values: A Lesbian Mother's Fight for Her Son* (New York: Prentice Hall Press, 1988), p. 229.

23. O'Hanlon, Katherine, "In a Family Way: Insemination 101," *The Advocate* 684, June 27, 1995, p. 49.

24. Lobenstine, p. 6.

25. Benkov; Lobenstine; Martin; Pies; Saffron.

26. O'Hanlan, Katherine, "Lesbian Health and Homophobia: Perspectives for the Treating Obstetrician/Gynecologist," *Current Problems in Obstetrics, Gynecology and Fertility* 18(4), July/August 1995, pp. 93–136.

27. Clendinen, "My Two Moms."

28. Burke, *Family Values*, pp. 32–33.

29. Rafkin, Louise, *Different Mothers* (Pittsburgh: Cleis Press, 1990); Saffron, Linda, *'What About the Children?'* (London: Cassell, 1996).

30. Ex., Raboy, Barbara, et al., "Mental Health Among Families with Children Conceived by Donor Insemination," ASRM 52nd Annual Conference, November 2–7, 1996, Boston.

31. Saffron, pp. 136–137.

32. Newman, Leslea, *Heather Has Two Mommies* (Boston: Alyson Publications, 1989); Abramchik, Lois, *Is Your Family Like Mine?* (New York: Open Heart, Open Mind, 1993). Order: 582 Fifth St., 2B, Brooklyn, NY 11215, $13; COLAGE, 2300 Market St., #165, San Francisco, CA 94114.

33. Hill, Kate, "Mothers by Insemination: Interviews," in *Politics of the Heart: A Lesbian Parenting Anthology*, ed. Pollack, Sandra, and Jeanne Vaughn (New York: Firebrand Books, 1987), p. 117.

34. Lobenstine, p. 16.

35. Burke, *Family Values*, p. 213.

36. Alpert, Harriet, *We Are Everywhere* (Freedom, CA: The Crossing Press, 1988); Arnup, Katherine, *Lesbian Parenting* (Charlottetown, P.E.I., Canada: Gynergy Books, 1995); Rizzo, Cindy, et al., *All the Ways Home* (Norwich, VT: New Victoria Publishers, 1995) (fiction); Wakeling, Louise, and Margaret Bradstock, *Beyond Blood* (Sydney, Australia: BlackWattle Press, 1995).

37. Greenberg, Keith Elliot. *Zack's Story: Growing Up with Same-Sex Parents* (Minneapolis, MN: Lerner Publications Co., 1996).

38. Martin, pp. 254–255.

39. Newman, Leslea, *Saturday Is Pattyday* (Norwich, VT: New Victoria Pub., 1993).

40. Benkov, pp. 227–240; Martin, pp. 245–257; Rafkin, Louise, *Different Mothers* (Pittsburgh: Cleis Press, 1990); Saffron.

41. Tortorilla, Toni, "On a Creative Edge," in *Politics of the Heart*, op. cit., p. 174.

42. Bernstein, *Yours, Mine, and Ours*.

43. Brown, Laurene and Marc, *Dinosaurs Divorce* (Boston: Little, Brown & Co., 1986); Pellegrini; Tax.

44. Bennett, Madeline, *Sudden Endings: Wife Rejection in Happy Marriages* (New York: William Morrow and Co.), 1991.

45. Teyber, Edward, *Helping Children Cope with Divorce* (New York: Lexington Books, 1992); Kalter, Neil, *Growing Up with Divorce* (New York: The Free Press, 1990); Blau, Melinda, *Families Apart: Ten Keys to Successful Co-Parenting* (New York: Perigee Books, 1994).

46. Kahn, Sandra, *The Ex-Wife Syndrome* (New York: Random House, 1990).

47. Cook, Jean Thor, *Room for a Stepdaddy* (Morton Grove, IL: Albert Whitman & Co., 1995).

48. For ex., Glazer, "Raising Biological and Adopted Children," in *The Long-Awaited Stork*; Simons; Melina.

49. Melina, pp. 143–144.

50. Cooper and Glazer; Gordon; Wickham.

51. Howe, James, *Pinky and Rex and the New Baby* (New York: Atheneum, 1993); Schnitter, Jane, *William Is My Brother* (Indianapolis: Perspectives Press, 1991); Wright, Susan, *Real Sisters* (Charlottetown, PEI, Canada: 1994).

52. Van Gulden, Holly, and Lisa Bartels-Rabb, *Real Parents, Real Children* (New York: Crossroad Pub. Co., 1993).

53. Johnston, *Taking Charge of Infertility*, p. 247.

54. Stein, Stephanie, *Lucy's Feet* (Indianapolis: Perspectives Press, 1992); Shreve, Susan, *Zoe and Columbo* (New York: Tambourine Books, 1995).

55. Pellegrini.

CHAPTER NINE

1. Hanson, p. 19.

2. Neufeld, pp. 3–4.

3. Zoldbrod, "The Emotional Distress of the Artificial Insemination Patient," p. 170.

4. Cook et al.

5. Menning, *Infertility*.

6. Fleming, Jeanne, "Infertility as a Chronic Illness," *RESOLVE National Newsletter*, December 1994, p. 5. © National RESOLVE. Reprinted with permission. Order the RESOLVE fact sheet "Infertility as a Chronic Illness and Stress Disorder."

7. Domar, Alice, et al., "The Psychological Impact of Infertility: A Comparison With Patients With Other Medical Conditions," *Journal of Psychosomatic, Obstetric and Gynacology* 14, Special Issue, 1993, pp. 45–52.

8. See all citations for Zoldbrod in the Bibliography.

9. Ferber, Geri, "An Empathy-Supporting Approach to the Treatment of Infertile Women," *Psychotherapy* 32(3), Fall 1995, p. 438.

10. Braverman, Andrea Mechanick, "Egg Donation: Psychological and Counseling Issues Surrounding Disclosure versus Privacy," in Seibel and Crockin, p. 283.

11. Neufeld, pp. 4–5.

12. Ibid.

13. Anonymous, "Reflections on a Donor Insemination Support Group."

14. Aronson, Diane, "The Globalization of Information" with sidebar "Questions to Ask About the Internet," *RESOLVE National Newsletter*, 22(2), Spring 1996, p. 2. © National RESOLVE; reprinted with permission.

CHAPTER TEN

1. Glahn, Sandi, "Webster Redefined." Reprinted with permission of the author.

2. Levy, Wendy, *Swim, Swim . . . : Talking to Sperm and Other Desperate Acts*, short film. Order: Gal Films, 5261 Miles Ave., Oakland, CA 94618, $29.95.

3. Mattes, p. 129.

Bibliography

Abrams, Tamar. "My Test-Tube Daddy," *Washingtonian* 29(6), March 1994, pp. 44–49, 114.

American Fertility Society. "Guidelines for Gamete Donation," *Fertility and Sterility* 59(2), Supplement 1, February 1993, pp. S1–9.

Andrew, Lori. *New Conceptions*. New York: Ballantine Books, 1984, pp. 142–178.

Annas, George. "Fathers Anonymous: Beyond the Best Interests of the Sperm Donor," *Child Welfare* 60(1), pp. 161–174.

Anonymous. "Resolving AID," *RESOLVE Newsletter*, April 1984, p. 4. © National RESOLVE. Reprinted with permission.

———. "Reflections on a Donor Insemination Support Group," *RESOLVE of NYC Newsletter*, June 1990, pp. 10–11.

———. "Confessions of a Sperm Donor," *Self* 13(11), November 1991, pp. 152–155, 180.

———. "Difficult Choice," *RESOLVE of NYC Newsletter*, May 1992, pp. 4, 7.

———. "One Donor's Story," *Washingtonian* 29(6), 1994, p. 49.

Anton, Linda Hunt. *Never to Be a Mother*. New York: HarperCollins, 1992.

Atallah, Lillian. "Report from a Test-Tube Baby," *New York Times Magazine*, April 18, 1976, pp. 16–17, 48–50.

Baran, Annette, and Reuben Pannor. *Lethal Secrets*. New York: Amistad Books, 1993 (Warner, 1989).

Beck, Peg. "Just Say No: Walking Away from Treatment," *RESOLVE of the Bay State Newsletter*, Summer 1993, pp. 3, 13.

Becker, Gay. *Healing the Infertile Family*. New York: Bantam Books, 1990.

Benkov, Laura. *Reinventing the Family: The Emerging Story of Lesbian and Gay Parents*. New York: Crown Publishers, 1994.

Bernstein, Anne. *Flight of the Stork*. Indianapolis: Perspectives Press, 1994.

———. *Yours, Mine, and Ours: How Families Change When Remarried Parents Have a Child Together*. New York: W. W. Norton & Company, 1989.

Berry, Joy. *Every Kid's Guide to Overcoming Prejudice and Discrimination*. Sebastopol, CA: Living Skills Press, 1987.

Blanchard, Amy. "Donor Insemination: Choosing an Identified or Anonymous Donor," *RESOLVE of Northern California Newsletter* 15(2), 1994, p. 10.

———. "Some Thoughts About Donor Insemination Practice," *RESOLVE of Northern California Newsletter* 14(1), 1993, pp. 14–15.

Blaustein, Muriel. *Play Ball, Zachary!* New York: Harper & Row, 1988.

Blizzard, Joseph. *Blizzard and The Holy Ghost, Artificial Insemination: A Personal Account.* London: Peter Owen Limited, 1977.

Bok, Sissela. *Secrets.* New York: Pantheon Books, 1982.

Bombardieri, Merle. "Childfree Decision-making." Order: RESOLVE.

———. *The Baby Decision.* New York: Rawson, Wade Publishers, 1981.

Bond, Pamela. "Three Months at a Time: Male Infertility and AID," *RESOLVE National Newsletter*, April 1984, p. 3. © National RESOLVE. Reprinted with permission.

Braverman, Andrea Mechanick, and Stephen Corson. "Factors Related to Preferences in Gamete Donor Sources," *Fertility and Sterility* 63(3), March 1995, pp. 543–549.

Brown, Margaret. "Whose Eyes Are These, Whose Nose?" *Newsweek*, March 7, 1994, p. 12. © 1994, Newsweek, Inc. All rights reserved. Reprinted by permission.

Carey, Benedict. "Sperm Inc.," *In Health* 5(4), 1991, pp. 50–56.

Cobb, Nathan. "Who Is My Donor Dad?" *The Boston Globe*, September 10, 1992, p. 85–87.

Cook, Rachel, Susan Golombok, Alison Bish, and Claire Murray. "Disclosure of Donor Insemination: Parental Attitudes," *American Journal of Orthopsychiatry* 56(4), October 1995, pp. 549–559.

Cooper, Susan, and Ellen Glazer. *Beyond Infertility: The New Paths to Parenthood.* New York: Lexington Books, 1994.

Curie-Cohen, Martin, Lesleigh Luttrell, and Sander Shapiro. "Current Practice of Artificial Insemination by Donor in the United States," *New England Journal of Medicine* (300)11, 1979, pp. 585–590.

Daniels, Ken. "Semen Donors: Their Motivations and Attitudes to Their Offspring," *Journal of Reproductive and Infant Psychology* 7(2), 1989, pp. 121–127.

——— and Gillian Lewis. "Donor Insemination: The Gifting and Selling of Semen," *Social Science and Medicine* 42(11), June 1996, pp. 1521–1536.

———, Gillian Lewis, and Wayne Gillett, "Telling Donor Insemination Offspring About Their Conception: The Nature of Couples' Decision-Making," *Social Science and Medicine* 40(9), May 1995, pp. 1213–1220.

———, et al. "Successful Donor Insemination and Its Impact on Recipients," *Journal of Psychosomatic Obstetrics and Gynecology* 17, September 1996, pp. 129–134.

Diamond, Ronny. "Secrecy vs. Privacy," *Adoptive Families*, September/October 1995, pp. 8–11. Reprinted by permission of OURS magazine, © 1995, Adoptive Families of America, 3333 Highway 100 North, Minneapolis, MN 55422.

Donor Conception Support Group of Australia, Inc. *Let the Offspring Speak.* ed. Caroline Lorbach, 1997, $37.50 U.S. including postage. Order: see Resources.

Drexler, Madeline. "The Baby Bank," *The Good Health Magazine, The Boston Globe*, October 7, 1990, pp. 9–11, 20–22.

Duka, Walter, and Alan DeCherney. *From the Beginning: A History of the American Fertility Society, 1944–1994.* Birmingham, AL: American Fertility Society, 1994. Order: American Society for Reproductive Medicine (see Resources).

Franz, Sherry. "The Sexual Legacy of Infertility: The Separation of Procreation and Recreation," *The Canadian Journal of Human Sexuality* 2(3), Fall 1993, pp. 105–106.

Fried, Stephen. "Baby Bank," *Redbook,* October 1992, pp. 108–111.

Gill, Mark Stuart. "The Genius Babies," *Ladies' Home Journal,* March 1995, pp. 76–82.

Glazer, Ellen. *The Long-Awaited Stork.* New York: Lexington Books, 1990.

———— and Susan Cooper. *Without Child.* New York: Lexington Books, 1988.

Golombok, Susan, Rachel Cook, Alison Bish, and Claire Murray. "Families Created by the New Reproductive Technologies: Quality of Parenting and Social and Emotional Development of the Children," *Child Development* 66(2), April 1, 1995, pp. 285–298.

Gonick, Larry, and Mark Wheelis. *The Cartoon Guide to Genetics.* New York: HarperPerennial, 1991.

Gordon, Elaine. *Mommy, Did I Grow in Your Tummy?* Santa Monica, CA: EM Greenburg Press, 1992.

Greil, Arthur. *Not Yet Pregnant.* New Brunswick, NJ: Rutgers University Press, 1991.

Guinan, Mary. "Artificial Insemination by Donor: Safety and Secrecy," *JAMA* 273(11), March 15, 1995, pp. 890–891.

Hancock, Marilyn. "When Dad's Only Name Is 'Anonymous Donor,'" *The Brockton Enterprise*, February 28, 1993, pp. 1, 17. Reprinted with permission.

Hanson, Michelle Fryer. *Infertility: The Emotional Journey.* Minneapolis: Deaconess Press, 1994.

Imber-Black, Evan. *Secrets in Families and Family Therapy.* New York: W. W. Norton & Company, 1993.

Infertility Research Trust. *My Story.* Sheffield, England: J. W. Northend Ltd, 1991. Order: Kris Probasco, LSCSW, 144 Westwood Dr., Liberty, MO 64068, $11.95 plus $3/book.

Johnston, Patricia. *Taking Charge of Infertility.* Indianapolis: Perspectives Press, 1994.

————. "The Guy on the Street and New-Tech Babies . . . Advice From the Trenches for Parents," and "What Should We Tell the Kids? Talking to Children about Our Infertility." Order: Perspectives Press, P.O. Box 90318, Indianapolis, IN 46290.

Karow, Armand. "Confidentiality and American Semen Donors," *International Journal of Fertility* 38, 1993, pp. 147–151.

Klock, Susan. "Psychological Aspects of Donor Insemination," *Infertility and Reproductive Medicine* 4(3), July 1993, pp. 456–469.

————, Mary Casey Jacob, and Donald Maier. "A Prospective Study of Donor Insemination Recipients: Secrecy, Privacy, and Disclosure," *Fertility and Sterility* 62(3), September 1994, pp. 477–484.

———— and Donald Maier. "Psychological Factors Related to Donor Insemination," *Fertility and Sterility* 56(3), September 1991, pp. 489–495.

Lang, Susan. *Women Without Children.* New York: Pharos Books, 1991.

Lawson, Carol. "Who Is My Daddy? Can Be Answered in Different Ways," *The New York Times,* August 5, 1993, p. C1.

Lerner, Harriet. *The Dance of Deception: Pretending and Truth-Telling in Women's Lives.* New York: HarperCollins, 1993.

LieberWilkins, Carole. "Sperm and Egg Donations: What You Need to Know." Audiotape of talk given at RESOLVE/Serono Symposium on October 1, 1994, in Los Angeles. Order: Professional Programs, P.O. Box 221466, Santa Clarita, CA 91322-1466, 805-255-7774, $8.75 plus $1.50.

———. "Talking to Children about Their Conception: A Parent's Perspective." Order from author: 1460 Westwood Blvd., Suite 204, Los Angeles, CA 90024.

Liebmann-Smith, Joan. *In Pursuit of Pregnancy: How Couples Discover, Cope With, and Resolve Their Fertility Problems.* New York: Newmarket Press, 1987. Reprinted with permission of Newmarket Press.

Lobenstine, Geoff. *Children, Lesbians and Men.* Alternative Families Project, 1994. Order: $10 check to Men's Resource Center, Alternative Families Project, 442 Warren Wright Road, Belchertown, MA 01007.

Mahlstedt, Patricia, and Dorothy Greenfeld. "Assisted Reproductive Technology with Donor Gametes: The Need for Patient Preparation," *Fertility and Sterility* (52)6, December 1989, pp. 908–914.

———, and Kris Probasco. "Sperm Donors: Their Attitudes Toward Providing Medical and Personal Information for Donor Offspring," *Fertility and Sterility* (56)4, October 1991, pp. 747–753.

Marsh, Margaret, and Wanda Ronner. *The Empty Cradle: Infertility in America from Colonial Times to the Present.* Baltimore: Johns Hopkins University Press, 1996.

Martin, April. *The Lesbian and Gay Parenting Handbook.* New York: HarperCollins, 1993.

Mason, Mary Martin. "Jennifer and Paula," in *The Miracle Seekers.* Indianapolis: Perspectives Press, 1987. Order: Adoptapes, 4012 Lynn Ave., Edina, MN, 55416, $14.95.

Mattes, Jane. *Single Mothers By Choice.* New York: Time Books/Random House, 1994.

May, Elaine Tyler. *Barren in the Promised Land.* New York: Basic Books, 1995.

McDaniel, Susan. "Within-Family Reproductive Technologies as a Solution to Childlessness Due to Infertility: Psychological Issues and Interventions," *Journal of Clinical Psychology* 1(4), 1985, pp. 301–308.

Melina, Lois. *Making Sense of Adoption.* New York: Harper & Row, 1989. (Treats DI as "semi-adoption.")

Menning, Barbara Eck. "Donor Insemination: the Psychosocial Issues," *Contemporary OB/GYN* 18(4), October 1981, pp. 155–172.

———. *Infertility: A Guide for the Childless Couple.* New York: Prentice Hall Press, 1988.

Morgentaler, Abraham. *The Male Body.* New York: A Fireside Book, 1993.

Nachtigall, Robert. "Secrecy: An Unresolved Issue in the Practice of Donor Insemination," *American Journal of Obstetrics and Gynecology* 168(6), June 1993, pp. 1846–1851.

———, et al., "Stigma, Disclosure, and Family Functioning among Parents of Children Conceived Through Donor Insemination," Fertility and Sterility, 68(1), July 1997, pp. 83–89.

Nelson, Pete. "Sperm Donors, The Guys Who Give," *New Woman*, November 1995, pp. 98–99, 141–143.

Neufeld, Marlene. "An Infertility Seminar: Congregate Pain and Hope," *Infertility Awareness* 8(5), August 1992, pp. 1, 3–5. © Infertility Awareness Association of Canada, Inc. Reprinted with permission of the author.

New South Wales Infertility Social Workers Group. *How I Began: The Story of Donor Insemination.* Ed. Julia Paul. Carlton, Victoria: The Fertility Society of Australia, 1988. Order: C/-ACTS GPO Box 2200, Canberra ACT 2601, Australia; phone (06) 257 3299.

Noble, Elizabeth. *Having Your Baby by Donor Insemination.* Boston: Houghton Mifflin, 1987.

Orenstein, Peggy. "Looking for a Donor to Call Dad," *New York Times Magazine*, June 18, 1995, pp. 28–35, 42, 50, 58.

Pellegrini, Nina. *Families Are Different.* New York: Holiday House, 1991.

Pfeffer, Naomi. *The Stork and the Syringe: A Political History of Reproductive Medicine.* Cambridge, England: Polity Press, 1993.

Pierce, Benjamin. *The Family Genetic Sourcebook.* New York: John Wiley & Sons, 1990.

Probasco, Kris. "How to Tell Children About Their Donor Conception: A Developmental Perspective." Order from author: 144 Westwood Dr., Liberty, MO 64068.

Raboy, Barbara. "Secrecy and Openness in Donor Insemination: A New Paradigm," *Politics and Life Sciences,* August 1993, pp. 191–192.

Riordan, Tom. "The Threat of DI," *RESOLVE of NYC Newsletter*, March 1994, pp. 1, 8.

——— and Joanna Feinman. "An Open Letter and Opposing View on DI," *RESOLVE of NYC Newsletter*, September 1994, p. 2.

Robertson, John. *Children of Choice: Freedom and the New Reproductive Technologies.* Princeton, NJ: Princeton University Press, 1994.

Robinson, Susan, and H. F. Pizer. *Having a Baby Without a Man.* New York: Simon and Schuster, 1985.

Rodrick, Stephen. "Upward Motility," *The New Republic* 210(10), May 16, 1994, pp. 9–10.

Roman, Mark. "Breaking the Genetic Silence," *Lear's*, January 1993, pp. 37–38.

Rosenberg, Helane, and Yakov Epstein. *Getting Pregnant When You Thought You Couldn't.* New York: Warner Books, 1993.

Rubin, Theodore Isaac. *Overcoming Indecisiveness.* New York: Avon Books, 1985.

Saffron, Lisa. *Challenging Conceptions: Planning a Family by Self-Insemination.* London: Cassell, 1994.

Salzer, Linda. *Surviving Infertility.* Rev. ed. New York: Harper Perennial, 1991.

Schaffer, Patricia. *How Babies and Families Are Made (There Is More Than One Way!).* Berkeley, CA: Tabor Sarah Books, 1988.

Schmidt, Robert. "Where Did I Get My Blue Eyes, Daddy?" *RESOLVE Newsletter*, December 1989, p. 9. © National RESOLVE. Reprinted with permission.

Schnitter, Jane. *Let Me Explain: A Story About Donor Insemination.* Indianapolis: Perspectives Press, 1995.

Schover, Leslie, Robert Collins, and Susan Richards. "Psychological Aspects of Donor Insemination: Evaluation and Follow-up of Recipient Couples," *Fertility and Sterility* 57(3), March 1992, pp. 584–589.

Seibel, Machelle, and Susan Crockin. *Family Building Through Egg and Sperm Donation.* Sudbury, MA: Jones & Bartlett, 1996.

Seligson, Susan. "Seeds of Doubt," © Susan V. Seligson, as first published in *The Atlantic Monthly*, March 1995, pp. 28, 30, 38–39.

Shapiro, Sander. "Strategies to Improve Efficiency of Therapeutic Donor Insemination," *Infertility and Reproductive Medicine Clinics of North America* 3(2), April 1992, pp. 469–485.

Shengold, Nina. "Maya's Story: A Single Mom's Tale of Artificial Insemination," *New Woman*, November 1995, pp. 100, 103, 144–145.

Simon, Norma. *All Kinds of Families.* Niles, IL: Albert Whitman & Company, 1976.

———. *Why Am I Different?* Morton Grove, IL: Albert Whitman & Company, 1976.

Simons, Harriet Fishman. *Wanting Another Child: Coping with Secondary Infertility.* New York: Lexington Books, 1995.

Smith, Holly. *My Parents Made Me in a Special Way: With Love and the Help of Donor Insemination*, 1997. Order: see New Reproductive Alternatives in Resources.

Tax, Meredith. *Families.* Boston: Little, Brown, 1981.

Topp, Karen. "Positive Reflections: Growing up as a DI Child," *The Canadian Journal of Human Sexuality* 2(3), Fall 1993, pp. 149–151.

Vercollone, Carol Frost, and Diane Clapp. "Donor Insemination: Facts and Decision-Making," 1995. © National RESOLVE. Reprinted with permission.

Webster, Harriet. "Secrets To Tell, Secrets To Keep," *Parents*, September 1988, pp. 115–116, 119–120.

Wickham, Narelle. *Where Did I Really Come From?* North Sydney, Australia: Allen & Unwin, 1992. Write to author for ordering info: Box 535, Dickson, ACT 2602, Canberra.

Zoldbrod, Aline. "The Emotional Distress of the Artificial Insemination Patient," *Medical Psychotherapy* 1, 1988, pp. 161–172.

———. *Getting Around the Boulder in the Road: Using Imagery to Cope with Fertility Problems*, 1990. Order booklet: Center for Reproductive Problems, 12 Rumford Road, Lexington, MA 02173, $8.50.

———. *Men, Women and Infertility: Intervention and Treatment Strategies.* New York: Lexington Books, 1993.

Index